Acupuncture Channels and Points

an interactive study and reference manual

DR JOAN CAMPBELL

Foreword by Dr Dianne M Connelly, PhD, MAc, MA
Chancellor, Tai Sophia Institute, Maryland, USA

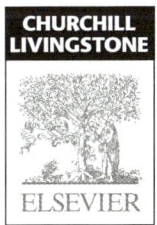

CHURCHILL LIVINGSTONE

ELSEVIER

Sydney   Edinburgh   London   New York   Philadelphia   St Louis   Toronto

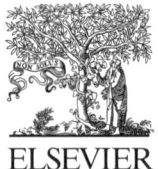

ELSEVIER

Churchill Livingstone
is an imprint of Elsevier

Elsevier Australia. ACN 001 002 357
(a division of Reed International Books Australia Pty Ltd)
Tower 1, 475 Victoria Avenue, Chatswood, NSW 2067

National Library of Australia Cataloguing-in-Publication Data

---

Campbell, Joan.

Acupuncture channels and points: an interactive study and
    reference manual / Joan Campbell.

Chatswood, NSW: Elsevier Australia, 2008.

978-0-72953-866-4 (pbk.)

Includes index.
Bibliography.

Acupuncture
Acupuncture points.

615.892

Publisher: Sophie Kaliniecki
Publishing Services Manager: Helena Klijn
Edited and indexed by Forsyth Publishing Services
Proofread by Pam Dunne
Illustrations by Nives Porcellato and Andrew Craig
Internal design and typesetting by Midland Typesetters
Cover design by Trina McDonald
Printed by 1010 Printing

Contents

Foreword

Dear reader,

There is an old saying — 'Give a person a fish and they eat for a day, teach a person to fish and they eat for a lifetime'.

Dr Joan Campbell is a teacher of 'fishing' when it comes to acupuncture — the ancient, ever-new practice of inserting needles into points along described channels.

I like that the root of the word manual — 'manus' — which means hands, and therefore Joan's manual is a 'hands-on' way to know our own aliveness through the tradition of this medicine … a human medicine carried by the Chinese, and like all medicine, an applied philosophy of being.

Her book is a way of saying 'here we are … memorise "that" we are here … now and now and now'. Use our body to know our body … we are that about which we study, and everything we say is something about our being here, a lifetime for each of us, however long.

The teaching ways of her manual evoke and allow learning to occur … with simple user-friendliness. You will see that each reader becomes a learner with ease, and that the old story of 'memorising' as a drudgery becomes a thrilling new practice. In this age of information, the bodied practices of learning are more important than ever … so we can turn information into knowledge that matters, and acquire wisdom that lasts a lifetime.

Dr Campbell is a person of ilk — a woman of substance. I know her first through the enormously high regard our intellectual colleagues have of her — in her innovative, rigorous and enlightened practices of medicine, inclusive of Eastern and Western thinking.

We can define medicine in many different ways. In my country, the United States of America, one definition that I find most profound is from the Cherokee. When one person does something for another, the other says: 'Thanks, that's a help'. So, a helping hand, a smile, a prescription, cooking a meal, teaching a class and drawing a distinction for living are all considered 'good medicine'.

I say this to you — whomever is reading this — as a way to reference Dr Joan Campbell, who knows, practises and teaches ways of being that give room for us to assist each other, to help see each other through in this journey of living and dying. Her being a doctor, a nurse, obstetric nurse, acupuncturist, teacher, wife, mother and grandmother are expressions of who she is as a great, glorious and gifted being of the human sort, loving and committed to humanity — the elders and the youngers.

'The way to do is to be', said Lao Tze, an ancient Chinese sage from the Dao De Ching. Joan is a virtuoso in recognising that all our doing comes from who we are. I am grateful for Joan's presence in my life. She lights up the philosophy upon which Chinese medicine is based, which then illumines the practices to which we have committed our lives.

I am honoured to be her colleague, friend and fellow traveller and I am continuously inspired by her. She is a gentle woman and a scholar. I trust my life in her hands and I am deeply happy to know her. You will be too.

Dianne M Connelly, PhD, MAc, MA
Dr Connelly has been a practitioner of traditional acupuncture since 1972, co-founder and chancellor of the Tai Sophia Institute (Maryland, USA) and international lecturer. She is the author of *Traditional Acupuncture: The Law of the Five Elements*, *All Sickness is Home Sickness*, and co-author of *Alive and Awake: Wisdom for Kids*. She is the mother of Blaize, Jade and Caeli, as well as grandmother to Tamar, Lennox and Rianna.

About the author

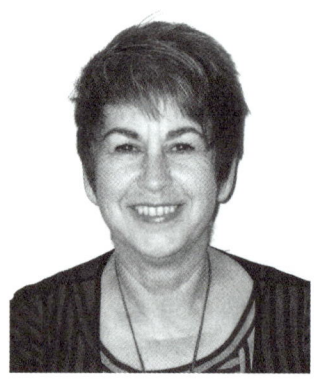

Dr Joan Campbell is an integrative health professional and registered medical practitioner specialising in acupuncture, working in her own well-established and successful medical practice in Auckland, New Zealand.

She has worked in medicine and allied fields since 1966, including as a registered nurse, medical doctor, GP obstetrician, psychologist (specialising in head injury), medical/traditional acupuncturist, university teacher and has an interest in homeopathic, nutritional and hormonal medicines.

Dr Campbell is a trained teacher and coordinator for the postgraduate and masters Traditional Chinese Medicine (TCM) programmes at the Auckland University of Technology, and pharmacology teacher at the New Zealand College of Chinese Medicine, Auckland.

Dr Campbell is:

- a former GP obstetrician who practised in Waitakere (1982–1990) and then specialist acupuncturist since 1990

- pharmacology teacher at the New Zealand College of Chinese Medicine, Auckland

- a member of the Australasian Integrative Medicine Association Inc (AIMA), New Zealand Institute of Acupuncture Inc (NZIA)

- a founding member of the New Zealand Qualifications Authority expert panel for acupuncture and the development of the National Diploma of Acupuncture and its revision

- coordinator of the application to government by the acupuncture profession for recognition of acupuncture as a profession under the *Health Practitioners Competency Assurance Act 2003*

- chairman of the New Zealand Acupuncture Standards Authority Inc (NZASA), which is recognised in statute as a registration authority for acupuncture treatment providers

- an organiser of numerous conferences and workshops for professional acupuncture groups and allied health professionals or professions; for example, the acupuncture satellite symposium of the 34th World Congress of the International Union of Physiological Societies, August 2001; and joint editor of the conference abstracts published in the International Congress series 1238, Excerpta Medica — Acupuncture, is there a physiological basis? (2002)

- a trustee of the Compassion in Healthcare Trust (NZ)

Dr Campbell is a wife to Graeme, mother to Janette and grandmother to Zachary.

Acknowledgments

Many people have contributed to the realisation of this manual. In particular I would like to thank the following people:

Diana Nash — friend, colleague, former teaching partner and co-founder of the first New Zealand Qualifications Authority approved private acupuncture teaching program in New Zealand (1993). The concepts of the diagrams in this book were originally developed jointly by us for that program and Di has kindly given permission for their continued use, modification and publication.

Neil Dingle — for drawing services relating to the 1990 diagrams.

Teachers — Dr Gerald Gibb, my first acupuncture teacher (Auckland, NZ); Dr Jiang (Nanjing University of Traditional Chinese Medicine, China); especially Dr Anita Cignolini (Milan, Italy) who gave me my first in-depth glimpse and understanding of TCM and spoilt me with her generosity and hospitality; and Myrene McLeod, a superb teacher of teachers.

Dianne Connelly — friend, respected colleague, co-founder and chancellor of the Tai Sophia Institute, Maryland, USA, which is now affiliated with Johns Hopkins University. Dianne brought her teaching gifts to NZ in 2000, shared with us her knowledge of 'Five Elements' and gave therapy to the acupuncturists attending the seminar. Thank you for your kind and loving foreword and for honouring the intrinsic value of the manual for student acupuncturists.

Jin Lan Yang — for providing the Chinese characters.

Students — past and present for their wisdom and their ability to challenge and extend my own knowledge.

Family — Graeme Campbell, my husband, and our beloved daughter Janette, for their strength and support, and being on the journey with me.

Vanessa Morgan — my practice manager, typist and superb formatter of documents, creative copywriter and chief sub-editor.

Bill Farrington — my orthopaedic surgeon who gave me back a functional left wrist and hand and the ability to continue to practise acupuncture.

Preface

In 1975 China intervened in my life. I spent 6 weeks in China with a University delegation during the last year of the Cultural Revolution — a time of great political turmoil, suffering and social chaos for many Chinese people. My husband, Graeme, was keen for us to be a part of the University delegation because of family ties to China through his second cousin, Rewi Alley. I took some persuading. However, the journey changed my life and my approach to medicine. In China, I was reintroduced to wholeness. Chinese medicine treated the whole person, not the disease; it understood the whole in order to treat the parts. I was back in a healing situation I felt content and comfortable with.

In 1989 I set out to work in Nanjing, 1 month after the killing of democracy students in Tianamen Square — a time of political re-education in China, a time of medical re-education for me. I had been working in General Practice since 1981 and doing Western style acupuncture since the early 1980s. A whole new world opened up for me with endless horizons. I was captivated. My practice would never be the same again.

I choose to work as a traditional Chinese acupuncturist with the traditional Chinese world view.

Medicine to me is about conversations and partnership between patient and therapist. Patients desire to be heard and understood, many want to be part of the healing partnership they have with their health professional, and most want to be considered an equal in the decision making for their health.

Chinese medicine has this to offer. The 'split' between man and nature and the 'split' of man into mind and body has never touched traditional Chinese philosophy. The classical Cartesian dichotomy which has paradoxically benefited and plagued modern Western medicine cannot be found in the theoretical constructs of Chinese medicine.

The person is treated, not the disease, and the disease simply is. There is only 'medicine' and our patients deserve to know which therapies work.

As a Western medical doctor, I have journeyed into Chinese medicine and found a therapeutic system of art and science that is unified in healing physically, mentally (emotionally) and spiritually, and which views individuals as whole beings with an inseparable body/mind, inseparable from the world and influenced by it.

By 'Chinese medicine' I mean the myriad and complex array of diagnostic, therapeutic and philosophical information developed in China since the dawn of time, studied and applied to humans and other animals, originating in the 'Daoist concepts of a universal cosmic energy (Dao) as the determining factor in life and health'.

The nature of Chinese medicine has been for me the fulfillment of a search for a sympathetic system of healing that embodies the inseparability of body and mind, spirit and matter, nature and man, philosophy and reality. It is a personal, subtle, gentle, yet highly technical medical system, which allows me to be close to the Chinese concept of 'qi', (crudely translated as 'energy' in Western equivalence), both my own and that of others.

The consequences and reasons for using it, teaching it and discussing it are twofold.

First, it works. It is commonly known to practitioners that Chinese medicine, including acupuncture, is capable of treating life's imbalances, not only those associated with the physical body, but also imbalances such as anxiety, neurosis, mania, depression, insomnia, and a whole range of psychological and emotional disorders.

Second, it is a humbling masterpiece of harmony, intricacy, and movement, which never ceases to engage me, fascinate me, intellectually challenge me, inspire me and intrigue me. It surrounds me in my work and life.

Dr Joan Campbell

Introduction

Acupuncture channels and points — an interactive study and reference manual

AIMS

1 To provide an interactive practical manual for students of acupuncture.

2 To provide a manual that is fun to use and enables channel theory, point location and body marking to be reinforced.

3 To enable students to understand and learn through drawing.

4 To provide students with a tool that will develop into a personal reference manual in their early years of practising acupuncture.

GENERAL

The manual is tried and tested, successful and authoritative. Moreover, it is a novel and modern system of learning that at once meets the educational and competency needs of today's health service, and yet honours and instils respect for the ancient tradition of Chinese acupuncture, including the use of Chinese pinyin names for channel points.

Learning the channel flows and point locations is time consuming and involves endless repetition. Students usually find their own ways to learn and recall this body of extensive information. However, with these diagrams, students are able to practise in their own time and reinforce and retain their channel knowledge.

By completing work sections on each channel students are given a framework for understanding the pathways of the channels, memorising points, identifying special points and learning their uses. It presents students with a methodical memory map of the primary channels and the extraordinary vessels.

In doing so, students interactively create their own study and reference text which will serve them throughout their early professional careers as acupuncturists.

Students are required to draw on sequential body outlines, progressively recording the flows and points of each channel. This discipline embeds in the mind and prompts an easily recalled system of channel flows, point notation and location.

This is not old-fashioned rote-learning of 365 points.

This is an enjoyable, and fun, system which complements all formal and self-directed learning of channel (*jing mai*) theory and practice — and teaches essential channel points for competent clinical practice.

How to get the most out of this manual

This fun-to-use manual reinforces channel marking and points.

Please read this section so you understand how to get the most out of this manual.

Enhance your learning by:

- practising your channel marking on a real body, working alone, in pairs or groups
- using supporting information and detailed point diagrams from acupuncture textbooks, such as *A Manual of Acupuncture* (Deadman, Al-Khafaji, Baker), *The Foundations of Chinese Medicine* (Maciocia) and *Chinese Acupuncture and Moxibustion* (chief editor Cheng Xinnong); see the reference list at the end of the manual
- doing the clinical case specific for each channel to reinforce your channel work.

This book focuses on:

- the main channel pathways and the extraordinary vessels
- the flow of *qi* in the main pathways (internal/external, superficial/deep)
- the points along the pathways
- the special points along the pathways.

Please note, this manual is *not* a point location textbook

This manual *does not* include:

- the luo-connecting channels (*luo mai*), divergent channels (*jing bie*), sinew channels (*jing jin*) or cutaneous regions (*pi bu*)
- point locations and functions
- measurements (proportional or hand cun).

What this manual covers

Chapters 1–14 cover the 12 primary channels, as well as two extraordinary vessels, Ren Mai and Du Mai.

Each chapter contains:

- a brief summary of the main pathway and other branches of the channel
  - 'main pathways' are the external representation of the channel you can access, which is drawn on the body where points are marked
  - 'other branches' are the deep or internal representation of the channel you cannot access, and are drawn on the body without points

- a list of point names and specific functions; that is, *yuan*-source points, *luo*-connecting points, *xi*-cleft points, influential points, the five *shu* (transporting) points, front-*mu* and back-*shu* points

Note: The points highlighted in bold are the most commonly used points, however different teaching programs will place an emphasis on different groups of points.

- a set of five progressive diagrams building a composite picture of a channel as each successive layer is added:
  1   the first is a blank body
  2   the second is a body showing the channel's internal and external branches and the flow of *qi*
  3   the third is a body showing the channel and the points and the flow of *qi*
  4   the fourth is a body showing the channel, points and the flow of *qi*
  5   the fifth is a composite body showing the channel, flow of *qi*, points and their names
- a case study using the points of the channel and any previous channels.

Chapter 15 covers the remaining **six extraordinary vessels**. This chapter contains the same elements as chapters 1–14, with two diagrams for each extraordinary vessel and case studies.

Appendix 1 provides a reference which shows you the physical structures and anatomical relationships of the body in four layers (the bones, the muscles, the blood vessels, the nerves).

Appendix 2 provides **case study answers**.

The **glossary** is on page xx and **references** are found at the end of the manual.

Tools

1   A piece of acetate film.

2   A fine-tip *non-permanent* marker of your choice.

3   Coloured pens and pencils, eraser etc.

4   An acupuncture textbook which has:
  –   the detailed point location information and diagrams
  –   methods of locating points (anatomical landmarks)
  –   proportional measurements and finger (cun) measurements (e.g. Deadman et al, Maciocia or other — see reference list).

5   Baroque music and a peaceful learning environment:
  –   Music stabilises mental, physical and emotional rhythms to attain a state of deep concentration and focus in which large amounts of content information can be processed and learned.
  –   Baroque music, such as that composed by Bach, Handel or Telemann — that is, 50 to 80 beats per minute — creates an atmosphere of focus that leads students into deep concentration in the alpha brainwave state.
  –   Studies have shown that learning vocabulary, memorising facts or reading to this music is highly effective.
  –   On the other hand, these same studies show that energising Mozart music assists in holding attention during sleepy times of the day and helps students stay alert while reading or working on projects — reference: http://www.newhorizons.org/strategies/arts/brewer.htm.

6   Use the glossary for any terms you are not familiar with.

7   Use the reference list for any additional texts to enhance your learning during the use of the manual.

How to use this manual

1   Read the beginning of each chapter and familiarise yourself with the channel you are about to work with, including the list of points for each channel.

2   Then, lay the acetate film over each body as required. Use your non-permanent marker to:

- **Body one**
  - Draw in the channel pathways (main and other branches), and draw in the flow of *qi* using directional arrows.
  - Draw in any anatomical markers you need — for example, bones, tendons, ligaments and so on — using the anatomical diagrams (see anatomical diagrams in Appendix 1).
  - Repeat this exercise as required until the channel location is firmly fixed in your mind.

- **Body two**
  - Draw in the channel points which are highlighted in bold on the point list, and show the flow of *qi*.
  - Draw in any anatomical markers you need — for example, bones, tendons, ligaments and so on — using the anatomical diagrams.
  - Repeat this exercise as required.

- **Body three**
  - Name each of the points using their pinyin and/or World Health Organization (WHO) numbering, and show the flow of *qi*.
  - Repeat this exercise as required until you can recall the names or numbers of the points and their location at random.

- **Body four**
  - Show the flow of *qi*, name the points and colour the appropriate special points: *yuan, luo, xi-cleft*, influential, front-*mu*, back-*shu* and the five *shu* (transporting).

For example:

yuan — blue	luo — red	xi-cleft — green	five shu — yellow
lower he-sea — orange	back-shu — purple	front mu-black	

Be consistent with your colours across all the channels

  - Repeat this exercise as required until you can recall the names or numbers of the points and their location at random.

- **Body five**
  - Check your work against the composite diagram.

Case studies

Read the case study and any additional textbooks as required. These case studies are drawn from 'real life' clinical practice.

Write your answers in pencil or on a separate sheet of paper. Check your answers in Appendix 2.

GUIDELINES TO POINT SELECTION

- **Acute**: choose points according to patterns, local/adjacent/distal points, empirical points, *xi*-cleft points, points on the affected channels and ah shi points.

- **Sub-acute**: choose points according to patterns, local/adjacent/distal points, empirical points, *biao li* relationships, *wu xing* dynamics, *he*-sea points, points on the affected channels and ah shi points.

The use of adjunct therapies like moxa and cupping should also be included where appropriate.

Please note:

1   The cases have been selected on the basis of reinforcing the functions of points on a specific channel.

2   The clinical cases progressively include the previous channels, for example the Lung Channel case study only uses points from the Lung Channel, whereas the Liver Channel case study includes points from all the 12 main channels.

   This enables the student to learn by combining points and reinforcing the point functions as they build their knowledge with each progressive channel case study. There is no standard point prescription. Many choices are given in the case study answers.

3   While the Lung Channel case study asks for points only from the Lung Channel, the author acknowledges that in clinical practice these may not be the 'best' points to use.

4   There are various diagnostic methods available. This manual uses only the 'Eight Principles' (*ba gang*) as a diagnostic tool to provide a consistent format for student acupuncturists to use.

Classification of Channels (Jing Mai) and the Circadian Rhythm of Qi

Channels are pathways which:

- are known as the *jing mai*
- circulate *qi* and *xue* (blood) to the entire body
- are related to the *zang fu* internally
- are made up of five parts.

Part one — the primary, main or regular channels usually referred to as the 12 channels and known as *jing mai*.

Part two — divergent channels which run with the primary channels and are called *jing bie*.

Part three — the sinew channels, or musculo-tendino channels, are known as the *jing jin*.

Part four — the eight extraordinary vessels, known as the *Qi Jing Ba Mai*, which are the deepest and most fundamental of the channel systems, linking our source *qi* to the universal *qi*. Two of the channels (Ren and Du) have points of their own and the remaining six vessels share points on the other channels. They interlink the primary channels to each other in the same way that reservoirs take water from canals and ditches during heavy rain.

Part five — connecting channels, known as the *luo mai*, which enmesh the body forming a network running transversely between the *jing mai*, and also the *fu luo*, or floating channels (Deadman et al refer to these as minute collaterals), which form small superficial branches on the surface of the body.

Note: The 12 cutaneous regions (*pi bu*) are not channels as such, but are skin regions overlying the network of main pathways, and are linked to them.

The Jing Mai

1 The *jing mai* can be classified according to their **nature** (i.e. *yin* or *yang*).

2 The *jing mai* can be classified based on the **location of their jing–well point** (the first or last point of the channel). Six channels start or end on the hand, and six start or end on the foot.
   Combining the two classifications gives us:

	Abbreviations	Pathway
3 Yin Channels of the Hand	LU, HT, PC	Chest to the hand
3 Yang Channels of the Hand	LI, SI, SJ/TE	Hand to the face
3 Yang Channels of the Foot	ST, BL, GB	Face to the foot
3 Yin Channels of the Foot	SP, KI, LR	Foot to the chest

3 The 12 main channels can be classified into **three categories or phases** according to their *yin* or *yang* energy. The Chinese have determined that some of the *yin* channels are more active or passive than others, in set phases, and similarly with the *yang* channels.
   The three groupings from active to less active (passive) are: maximum/supreme phase, equilibrium phase, minimum/lesser phase.

This can be tabulated as follows:

Energetic phase	Yin Channels	Yang Channels
Hand maximum	Lung	Small Intestine
Hand equilibrium	Pericardium	Large Intestine
Hand minimum	Heart	San Jiao/Triple Energiser
Foot maximum	Spleen	Bladder
Foot equilibrium	Liver	Stomach
Foot minimum	Kidney	Gall Bladder

Note: Deadman et al refer to these Energetic Phases as Supreme/Absolute and Brightness/Lesser.

If the three classifications are combined, we arrive at one classical arrangement that denotes the nature of the channels in greater detail:

The 12 Jing Mai in classical arrangement and terminology

1.	The Lung Channel of Hand	Taiyin (LU)*	Yin maximum
2.	The Large Intestine Channel of Hand	Yangming (LI)	Yang equilibrium
3.	The Stomach Channel of Foot	Yangming (ST)	Yang equilibrium
4.	The Spleen Channel of Foot	Taiyin (SP)	Yin maximum
5.	The Heart Channel of Hand	Shaoyin (HT)	Yin minimum
6.	The Small Intestine Channel of Hand	Taiyang (SI)	Yang maximum
7.	The Bladder Channel of Foot	Taiyang (BL)	Yang maximum
8.	The Kidney Channel of Foot	Shaoyin (KI)	Yin minimum
9.	The Pericardium Channel of Hand	Jueyin (PC)	Yin equilibrium
10.	The San Jiao/Triple Energiser Channel of Hand	Shaoyang (SJ/TE)	Yang minimum
11.	The Gall Bladder Channel of Foot	Shaoyang (GB)	Yang minimum
12.	The Liver Channel of Foot	Jueyin (LR)	Yin equilibrium

Note: See end of Glossary section for Table of Acupuncture Channel Abbreviations (Codes).

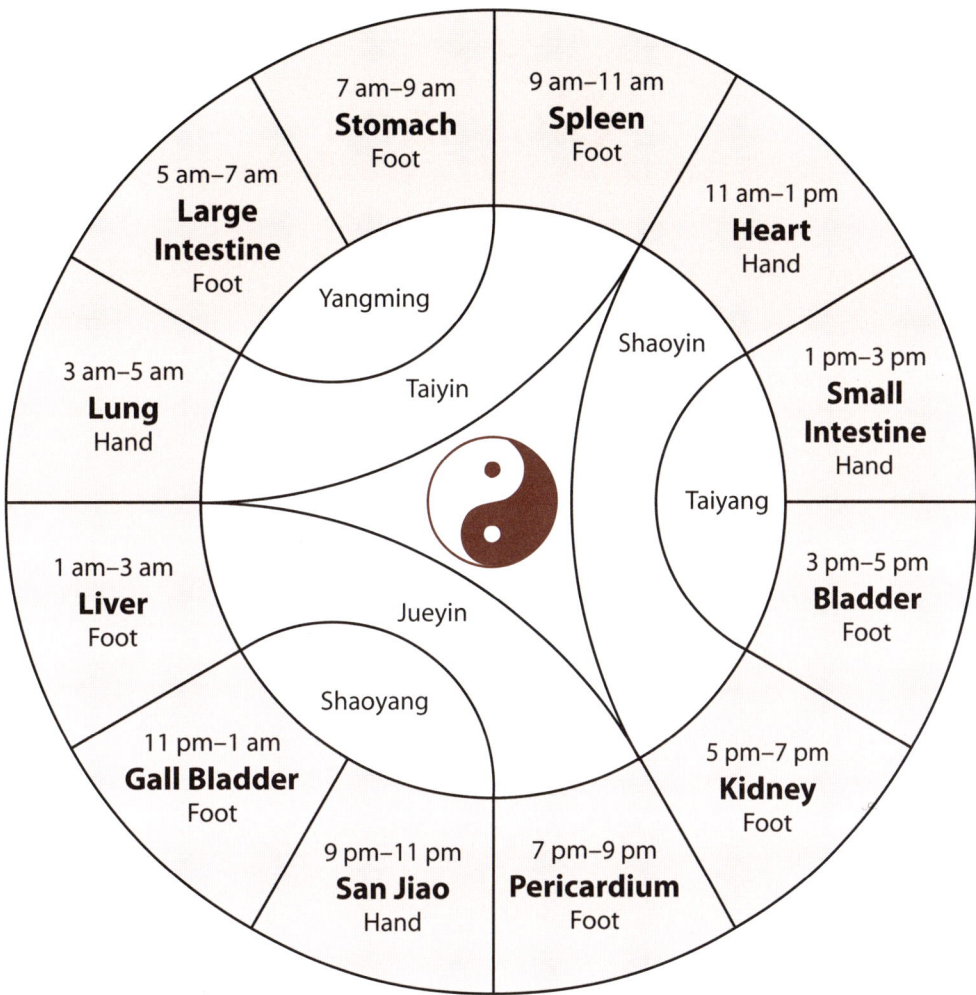

Timely progression of Qi through the body
Yin/Yang partners and Six Channel Theory

The Chinese have determined that the *qi* flows in an uninterrupted cycle from one channel to another in a **continuous and set pattern**.

The flow commences in the Lung Channel and terminates with that of the Liver, only to flow back to the Lung and start all over again.

The cycle takes 24 hours, starting at 3 a.m. with the flow in the Lung Channel, and is called the circadian rhythm of *qi*.

Glossary

Abbreviations

The channel abbreviations are approved by the World Health Organization (WHO). For example:

- Kidney = KI
- Stomach = ST
- Bladder = BL etc.

Chinese pinyin names are given in brackets for each definition.

Acupuncture (*zhen jiu*)

The word acupuncture means to puncture with a needle and comes from Latin:

- the noun 'acus', needle
- the verb 'punctare', to puncture.

In Traditional Chinese Medicine it is named '*zhen jiu*' 针灸 meaning needle and moxa (the use of burning a Chinese herb, Artemesia Vulgaris).

Today acupuncture means the insertion of fine, sterile, stainless steel needles into specific acupuncture points along channels, based on the clinical diagnosis for a particular individual.

Acupuncture is part of Traditional Chinese Medicine. It is 'grounded in conscientious observation of phenomena …' and 'has a body of knowledge with standards that allow practitioners to describe, diagnose and treat illness' (Vincent & Richardson, Pain 1996).

> In 1979 the World Health Organization held an interregional seminar in which it defined a number of diseases for which acupuncture could be considered to be potentially helpful. These include the treatment of acute infections and inflammation, dysfunction of the autonomic nervous system, several cardiovascular diseases, asthma, tinnitus, drug abuse, mood and behaviour disorders and various central and peripheral neurological diseases.
>
> (Sato, Li, Campbell 2002, vii)

Biao li (*biao li*)

Biao and *li* are two of the eight principles which determine the relative location of illness and the direction of the development of disease.

Biao means the exterior manifestations of things and events.

Li means interior syndromes.

Bi Syndrome (*bi*)

Bi means 'obstruction' which:

- is a syndrome of the channels rather than the internal organs
- presents as pain, soreness, swelling, distension, heaviness or numbness of muscles, tendons and joints

- is caused by invasion of external climatic pathogenic factors: *wind*, *cold* and *damp*, which lead to stasis of *qi* and *xue* (blood) in the channels and collaterals.

Bi is classified into four types:

1 Wandering *bi* in which pathogenic *wind* predominates.

2 Painful *bi* in which pathogenic *cold* predominates.

3 Fixed *bi* in which pathogenic *damp* predominates.

4 Febrile *bi* in which *wind*, *cold* and *damp*, over time, transform into *heat*.

Blood (*xue*)

Blood is a material substance which:

- moistens and nourishes the entire body through circulation
- is the mother of *qi*
- is inseparable from *qi* — *qi* infuses life into *xue* and without *qi*, *xue* would not flow
- is a *yin* fluid
- moves and circulates with *qi*.

Channels (*jing mai*)

Channels are composed of any of the main pathways of *qi* and *xue*. Distinction is made between the 12 primary channels and the 8 extraordinary vessels.

(See introduction for further information.)

Cupping (*ba guan fa*)

A method of treatment which applies suction to the body using cups, which:

- removes stagnant *qi* and *xue*
- promotes blood and *qi* circulation
- draws to the surface and expels pathogenic factors (e.g. *wind* obstructing the channels)
- dispels *damp*
- relieves pain by drawing blood into muscle
- relieves contracture by drawing blood into ligaments and tendons
- adjusts and enhances *zang fu* functions
- treats *bi* syndrome pain.

Jing (*jing*)

Jing is translated as 'essence' which:

- has no equivalent in western medicine
- is responsible for determining physical growth and development, reproduction and maintenance of life
- produces marrow, which then produces bone marrow, and also fills the spinal cord and brain
- is a *yin* substance
- is the root of life.

Jin ye (*jin ye*)

Jin ye embraces all normal fluid substances of the body, other than blood, which:

- has two types
  - *jin* liquid; for example, watery fluids moistening mucous membranes
  - *ye* humour; for example, thick turbid fluids (e.g. synovial fluid)
- are *yin* in nature.

Moxibustion (*jiu fa*)

A method of treatment which burns moxa (dried material from the herb mugwort, Artemesia Vulgaris) to apply heat to points and areas on the body, either directly or indirectly, which:

- stops bleeding by warming channels
- cools heat and dispels pathogenic factors
- moves stagnant blood and *qi* in affected areas and channels
- facilitates smooth *qi* and blood circulation
- warms and tonifies *qi*
- strengthens *yang qi* and prevents collapse
- nourishes and invigorates blood
- disperses *cold* and expels *wind*
- relieves pain
- can be used locally or systemically.

Qi (*qi*)

Qi is the vital force of life which:

- has countless forms as it moves and transforms
- is the material substrate of the universe
- is the material and spiritual substrate of human life
- is a primordial impulse which stands at the origin of the universe and creates all the phenomena within it
- is the birth and death of life
- is *yang* in nature
- is the western concept of energy (mc_2).

Shen (*shen*)

Shen, said to be stored by the heart, is an elusive concept which:

- is best translated as 'spirit' or 'mind'
- is the capacity of the mind to form ideas, think, feel and respond
- is the desire and force of the personality to live life, to be conscious and alert during the day and inactive during sleep
- is the ability to think, discriminate and choose appropriately
- is seen as the sparkle in the eyes, and the spring in the step.

Stagnant (*zhi*)

Affected by stagnation, *zhi*:

- refers to the circulation of the fundamental substances *qi* and *xue*
- leads to blockage in channels when the stagnation is chronic.

Stasis (*yu*)

Stasis is sluggish movement, especially of blood.

Xie Qi (*xie qi*)

Xie qi is pathogenic or 'evil' *qi* which:

- refers to any external illness–causing factor
- is usually related to the six climatic factors: *wind, cold, fire, damp, summer heat* and *dryness*.

Yin Yang (*yin and yang*)

Yin and *Yang* are the two fundamental forces in the universe which:

- are ever opposing, independent and interchanging
- sustain and complement each other
- are present in every aspect of life; for example, male is *yang*, female is *yin*, sunshine is *yang*, shadow is *yin* etc.

Zang fu (*zang fu*)

Zang fu are the internal organs which are divided into *zang* and *fu*:

- *zang* are *yin* solid organs — heart, liver, spleen, lung, kidney, pericardium — which transform and store vital substances in the body
- *fu* are *yang* hollow organs — small intestine, gall bladder, stomach, large intestine, bladder, san jiao — which are mainly involved in transporting nutrients into, or waste out of, the body.

TABLE OF ACUPUNCTURE CHANNEL ABBREVIATIONS (CODES)

Channel	Campbell	WHO 1991	Deadman et al	Maciocia
Lung	LU	LU	LU	LU
Large Intestine	LI	LI	L.I.	L.I.
Stomach	ST	ST	ST	ST
Spleen	SP	SP	SP	SP
Heart	HT	HT	HE	HE
Small Intestine	SI	SI	SI	S.I.
Bladder	BL	BL	BL	BL
Kidney	KI	KI	KID	KI
Pericardium	PC	PC	P	P
San Jiao	SJ	TE	SJ	T.B.
Liver	LR	LR	LIV	LIV
Gall Bladder	GB	GB	GB	G.B.
Ren Mai	Ren	CV	REN	Ren
Du Mai	Du	GV	DU	Du
Chong Mai	Chong	TV		
Dai Mai	Dai	BV		
Yang Qiao Mai	Yang Qiao	Yang HV		
Yin Qiao Mai	Yin Qiao	Yin HV		
Yang Wei Mai	Yang Wei	Yang LV		
Yin Wei Mai	Yin Wei	Yin LV		

References

Academy of Traditional Chinese Medicine, 1975. An Outline of Chinese Acupuncture. Foreign Languages Press, Peking, China

Anatomical Atlas of Chinese Acupuncture Points, 1990. Shandong Science and Technology Press, Jinan, China

Anderson J E, 1978. Grant's Atlas of Anatomy, 7th edn. Williams and Wilkins Co, USA

Brewer C, 1995. Music and Learning: Integrating Music in the Classroom. LifeSounds Educational Services, Bellingham, Australia

Cheng Xinnong (chief ed.), 1987. Chinese Acupuncture and Moxibustion. Foreign Languages Press, Beijing, China

Deadman P, Al-Kafaji M, Baker K, 2006. A Manual of Acupuncture. Journal of Chinese Medicine Publications, England

Ding L, 1991. Acupuncture Meridian Theory and Acupuncture Points. Foreign Languages Press, Beijing, China

Maciocia G, 2006. The Foundations of Chinese Medicine. Churchill Livingstone, Edinburgh, UK

Matsumoto K, Birch S, 1986. Extraordinary Vessels. Paradigm Publications, Massachusetts, USA

Netter F H, 1987. The Ciba Collection of Medical Illustrations, volume 8, Musculoskeletal System. Ciba-Geigy Corporation, Sumnit, New Jersey, USA

O'Connor J, Bensky D (translators and eds), 1981. Acupuncture: A Comprehensive Text, Shanghai College of Traditional Medicine. Eastland Press, Seattle, USA

Ross J, 1995. Acupuncture Point Combinations: The Key to Clinical Success. Churchill Livingstone, London, UK

Sato A, Li P, Campbell JL (eds), 2002. Acupuncture — is there a physiological basis? Satellite Symposium of the 34th World Congress of the IUPS. Excerpta Medica International Congress Series 1238. Elsevier Science, The Netherlands

State Standard of the People's Republic of China: The Location of Acupoints, 1990. Foreign Languages Press, Beijing, China

Vincent C A & Richardson P H, 1986. The evaluation of therapeutic acupuncture: concepts and methods. Pain, 24:1–13

Wiseman N, Ye F, 1998. A Practical Dictionary of Chinese Medicine, 2nd edn. Paradigm Publications, Brookline, Massachusetts, USA

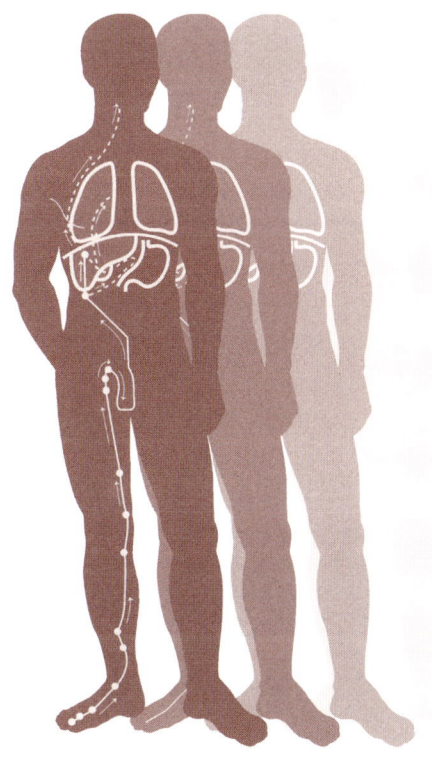

Chapter One

THE LUNG CHANNEL OF HAND TAIYIN

手太阴肺经

The Lung Channel of Hand Taiyin is *biao li* partnered with the Large Intestine Channel and paired with the Spleen Channel according to six channel theory.

The use of the Lung Channel is based on knowing the functions and indications of the Lung Channel points and the pathophysiology of the lung as a *zang*.

The Lung Channel connects with the following zang fu:

Stomach   Large Intestine   Lung

The main pathway:

- emerges at Zhongfu LU1 and ascends one rib space below the lateral extremity of the clavicle

- runs anteriorly across the shoulder and descends along the antero-lateral aspect of the upper arm, lateral to the Pericardium and Heart Channels

- passes through the anti-cubital fossa and along the antero-lateral aspect of the forearm, lateral to the Pericardium and Heart Channels

- follows the lateral border of the radial artery at the wrist

- crosses the thenar eminence at the junction between the pink and white skin and ends at the radial side of the thumb nail at Shaoshang LU11

- a branch leaves the main channel at the radial styloid (Lieque LU7) which travels directly to the radial side of the tip of the index finger where it links with the Large Intestine Channel of Hand Taiyang at Shangyang LI1.

The other branch:

- begins in the stomach descending deep into the large intestine

- returns upward over the gastro-oesophageal sphincter of the stomach

- passes through the diaphragm, enters and spreads into the lung

- ascends to the clavicular notch and throat

- then passes downwards across the upper chest to emerge 1 cun inferior to the lateral extremity of the clavicle at Zhongfu LU1.

The Lung Channel has no connections with other primary channels at any points on the body.

THE LUNG CHANNEL POINTS

WHO number	Pinyin	Name	Specific functions
LU1	**Zhongfu**	Central Treasury	Front-Mu
LU2	**Yunmen**	Cloud Gate	
LU3	**Tianfu**	Celestial Treasury	
LU4	**Xiabai**	Guarding White	
LU5	**Chize**	Cubit Marsh	He-Sea*5
LU6	**Kongzui**	Collection Hole	Xi-Cleft
LU7	**Lieque**	Broken Sequence	Luo-Connecting, Confluent Ren Mai
LU8	**Jingqu**	Channel Ditch	Jing-River*4
LU9	**Taiyuan**	Great Abyss	Shu-Stream*3, Yuan-Source, Influential Point of Vessels
LU10	**Yuji**	Fish Border	Ying-Spring*2
LU11	**Shaoshang**	Lesser Shang	Jing-Well*1

* The 5 Shu points of the Yin Channels:

    1 = wood

    2 = fire

    3 = earth

    4 = metal

    5 = water

Note: The 11 points highlighted in bold are provided on the composite diagram for this channel (the fifth diagram).

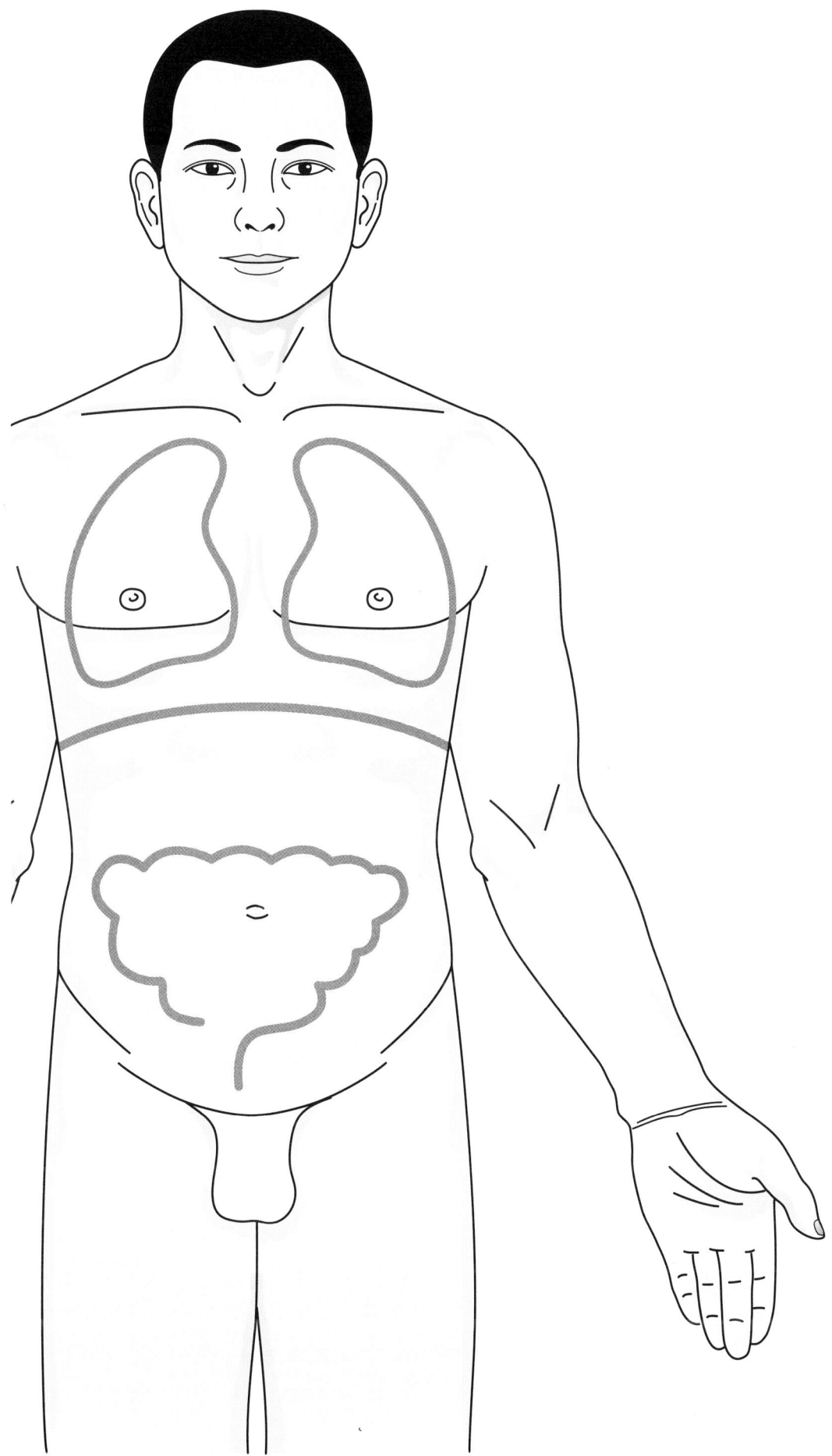

Figure 1.1 Lung Channel — Stage 1

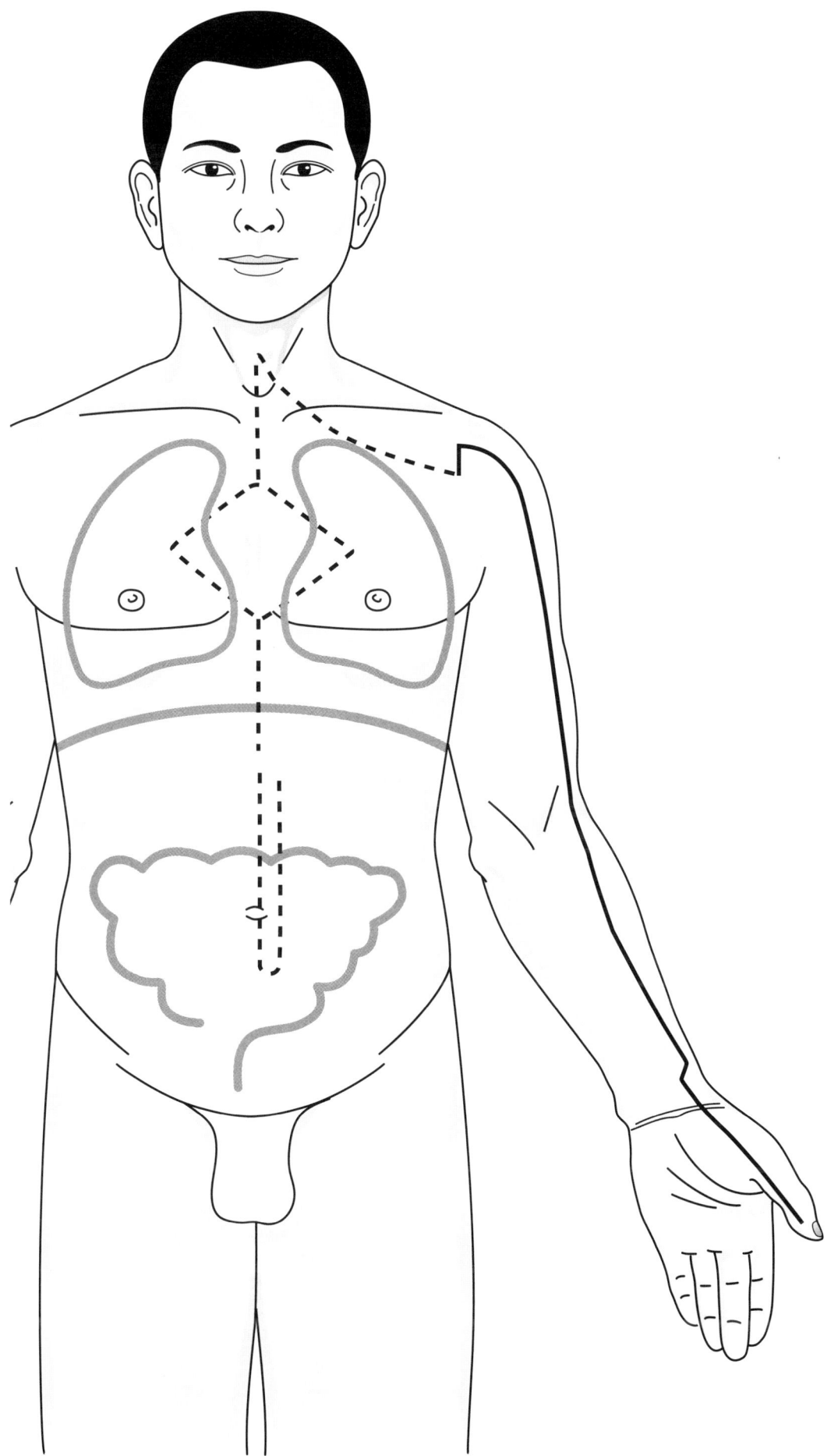

Figure 1.2 Lung Channel — Stage 2

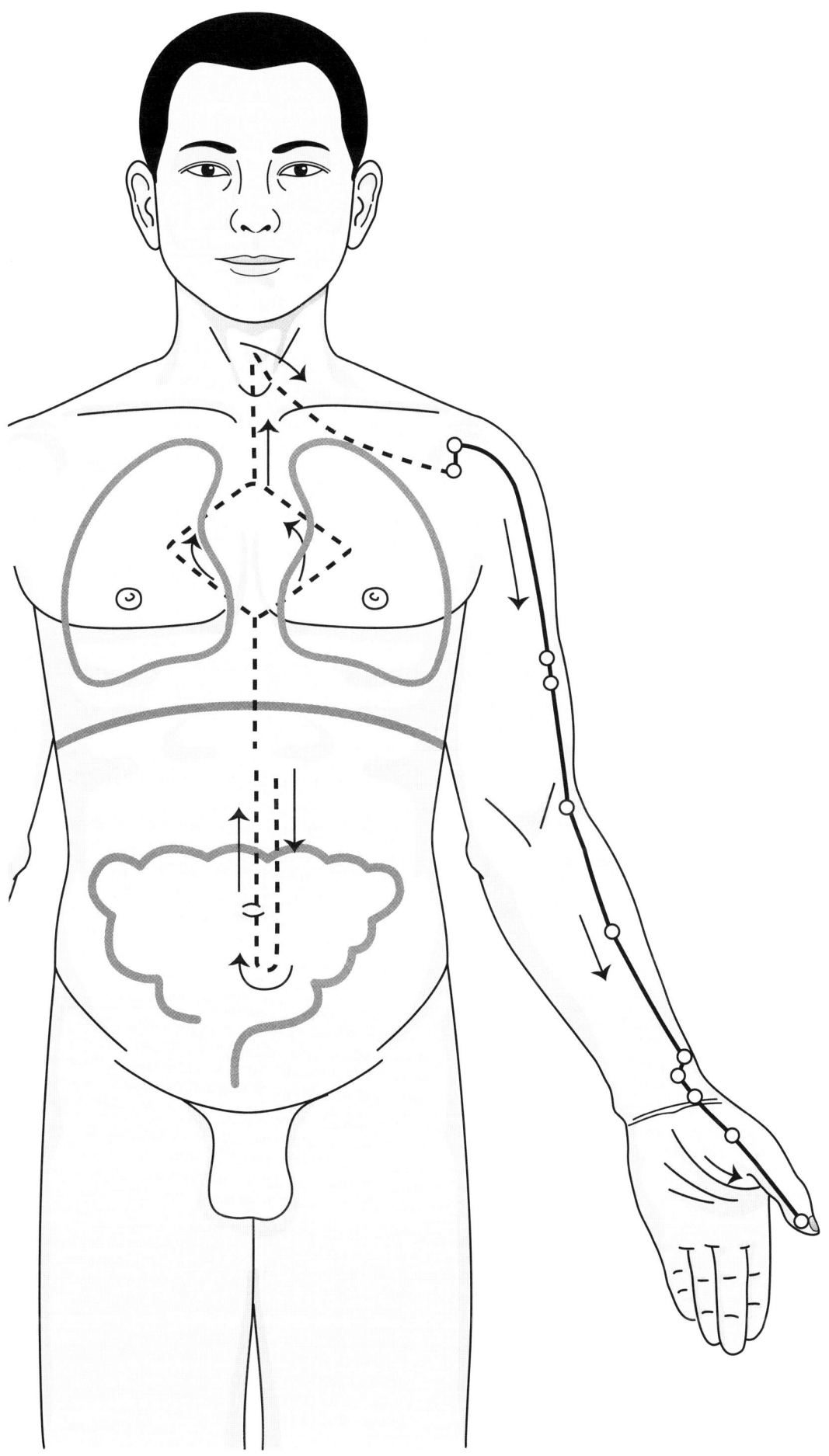

Figure 1.3 Lung Channel — Stage 3

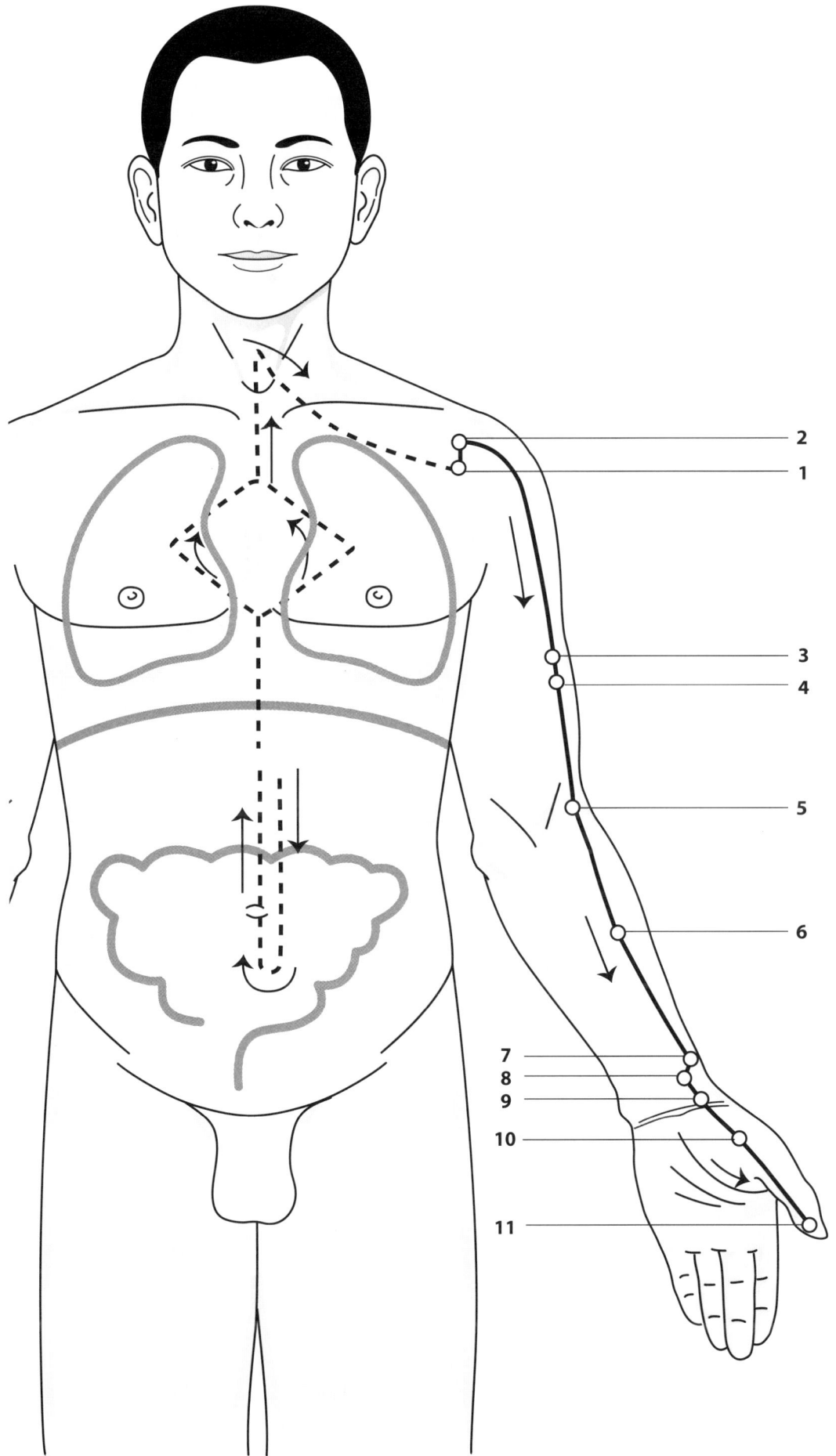

Figure 1.4 Lung Channel — Stage 4

yuan — blue	
luo — red	
xi-cleft — green	
five shu — yellow	
lower he-sea — orange	
back-shu — purple	

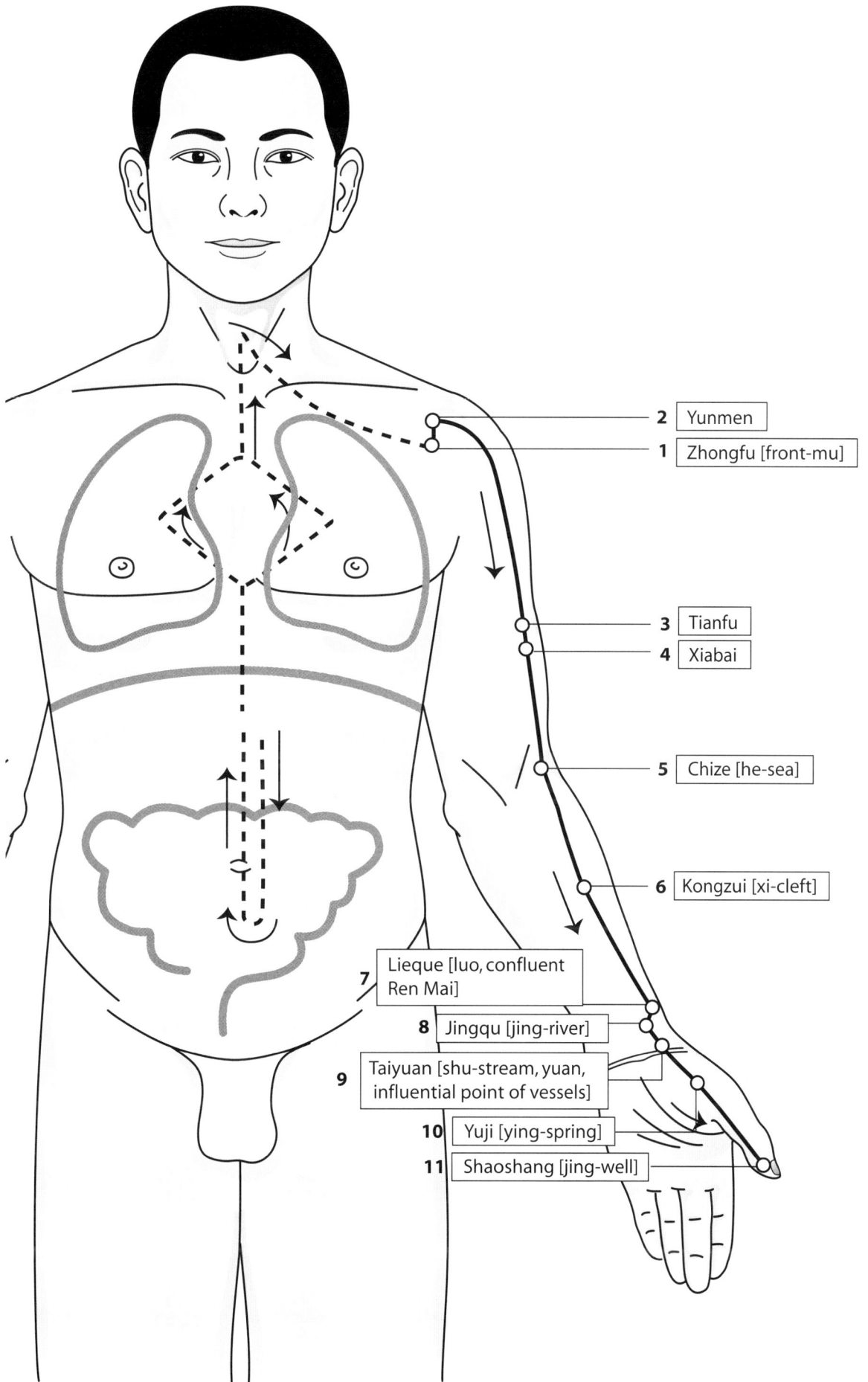

2 | Yunmen
1 | Zhongfu [front-mu]
3 | Tianfu
4 | Xiabai
5 | Chize [he-sea]
6 | Kongzui [xi-cleft]
7 | Lieque [luo, confluent Ren Mai]
8 | Jingqu [jing-river]
9 | Taiyuan [shu-stream, yuan, influential point of vessels]
10 | Yuji [ying-spring]
11 | Shaoshang [jing-well]

Figure 1.5 Lung Channel — Stage 5

THE LUNG CHANNEL — CASE STUDY

Miss MP, 26 year old receptionist

Miss MP presents to her health professional complaining of a cough, shivers, sneezing, slight fever, generalised head and body aches, aversion to cold, runny nose with clear nasal discharge and a lack of perspiration. These symptoms have been present for 24 hours.

QUESTIONS

Circle or write your answers as required.

1   Is this an external or internal disorder?

2   If external:
(a) Is it due to heat or cold?

(b) Are there symptoms of wind, dampness or dryness?

(c) Is it acute, chronic or a mixed condition?

3   If internal:
(a) Is it due to deficiency or excess?

(i) If deficient, is it: qi, blood, jin ye, yin or yang?

(ii) If excess, is it: stagnant qi, stagnant blood, damp/phlegm, rebellious qi, rising liver yang, empty fire etc?

(b) Is it due to cold or heat?

(c) Which zang fu are affected?

(d) Which channels are affected?

4   What might the pulse feel like?
Describe: pulse rate, rhythm, depth, shape and strength.

5 What might the tongue look like?
Describe:
– tongue body (colour, shape, thickness)
– tongue coating (moisture, colour, thickness, distribution, root).

6 What is the Chinese diagnosis?
Where appropriate, discuss the root (ben), the presenting symptoms (biao) and the five phase/wu xing dynamics (the relationship between and among the zang fu organs under syndromes of imbalance or disease).

7 What is your treatment principle?

8 What points would you use and why? Include adjunctive therapy such as moxa or cupping, if appropriate.
(Use only points on the Lung Channel.)

Chapter Two

THE LARGE INTESTINE CHANNEL OF HAND YANGMING

手阳明大肠经

The Large Intestine Channel of Hand Yangming is *biao li* partnered with the Lung Channel and paired with the Stomach Channel according to six channel theory.

The use of the Large Intestine Channel is based on knowing the functions and indications of the Large Intestine Channel points and the pathophysiology of the large intestine as a *fu*.

The Large Intestine Channel connects with the following zang fu:

Large Intestine   Lung

The main pathway:

- starts from the radial edge of the tip of the index finger at Shangyang LI1

- runs upward along the radial side of the index finger passing through the interspace between the first and second metacarpal bones

- dips into the depression between the tendons of extensor pollicus longus and brevis

- continues up the lateral anterior aspect of the forearm to the lateral side of the elbow

- ascends the lateral anterior aspect of the upper arm to the highest point of the shoulder joint

- crosses behind the shoulder along the border of the acromion between the scapular spine and the lateral extremity of the clavicle

- travels in a medial direction to just below the spinous process of the seventh cervical vertebra at Dazhui Du14 and then descends to the supraclavicular fossa (dividing into internal and external branches)

- the external branch continues up the lateral aspect of the neck, passes along the lower jaw entering the gums of the bottom teeth

- at the midline it curves back around the lips and crosses its partner channel at the philtrum, each partner channel passing to the opposite side of the nose (left channel to the right side of the nose and vice versa)

- joins with an internal branch of the Stomach Channel of Foot Yangming at Yingxiang LI20.

The other branch:

- begins and descends from the supraclavicular fossa
- connects with the lung
- descends through the diaphragm
- enters into the large intestine
- the 'Spiritual Pivot' states that the channel continues descending from the large intestine to Shangjuxu ST37.

The Large Intestine Channel connects with other primary channels at various points on the body, specifically the Stomach, Small Intestine, Du Mai, Ren Mai and Gall Bladder (not always shown in diagrams) Channels.

THE LARGE INTESTINE CHANNEL POINTS			
WHO number	Pinyin	Name	Specific functions
LI1	**Shangyang**	Shangyang	Jing-Well*1
LI2	**Erjian**	Second Space	Ying-Spring*2
LI3	**Sanjian**	Third Space	Shu-Stream*3
LI4	**Hegu**	Union Valley	Yuan-Source
LI5	**Yangxi**	Yang Ravine	Jing-River*4
LI6	**Pianli**	Veering Passageway	Luo-Connecting
LI7	**Wenliu**	Warm Dwelling	Xi-Cleft
LI8	**Xialian**	Lower Ridge	
LI9	**Shanglian**	Upper Ridge	
LI10	**Shousanli**	Arm Three Li	
LI11	**Quchi**	Pool at the Bend	He-Sea*5
LI12	Zhouliao	Elbow Bone-Hole	
LI13	Shouwuli	Arm Five Li	
LI14	**Binao**	Upper Arm	
LI15	**Jianyu**	Shoulder Bone	
LI16	**Jugu**	Great Bone	
LI17	**Tianding**	Celestial Tripod	
LI18	**Futu**	Protuberance Assistant	
LI19	Kouheliao	Grain Bone-Hole	
LI20	**Yingxiang**	Welcome Fragrance	

* The 5 Shu points of the Yang Channels:

    1 = metal
    2 = water
    3 = wood
    4 = fire
    5 = earth

Note: The 17 points highlighted in bold are provided on the composite diagram for this channel (the fifth diagram).

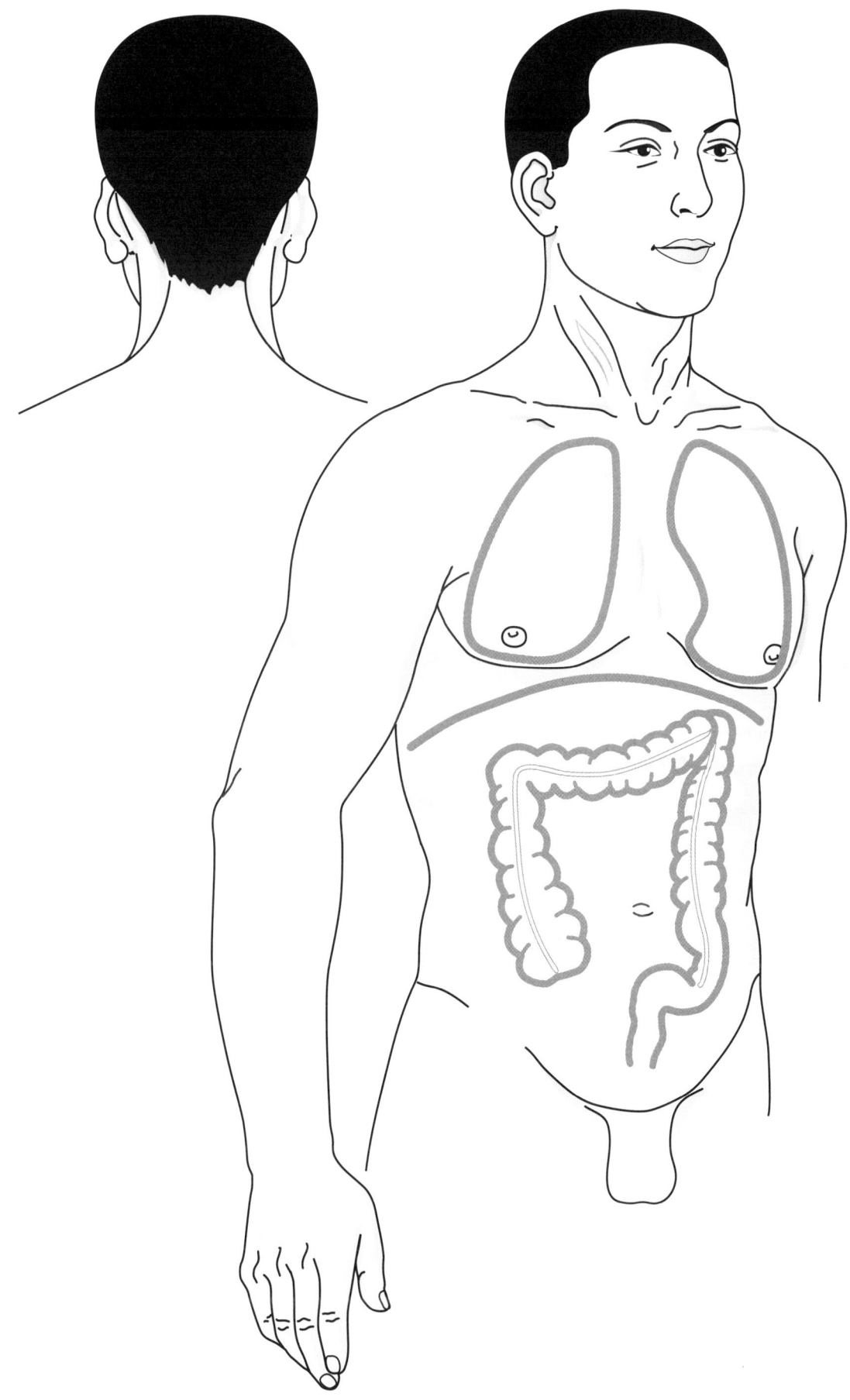

Figure 2.1 Large Intestine Channel — Stage 1

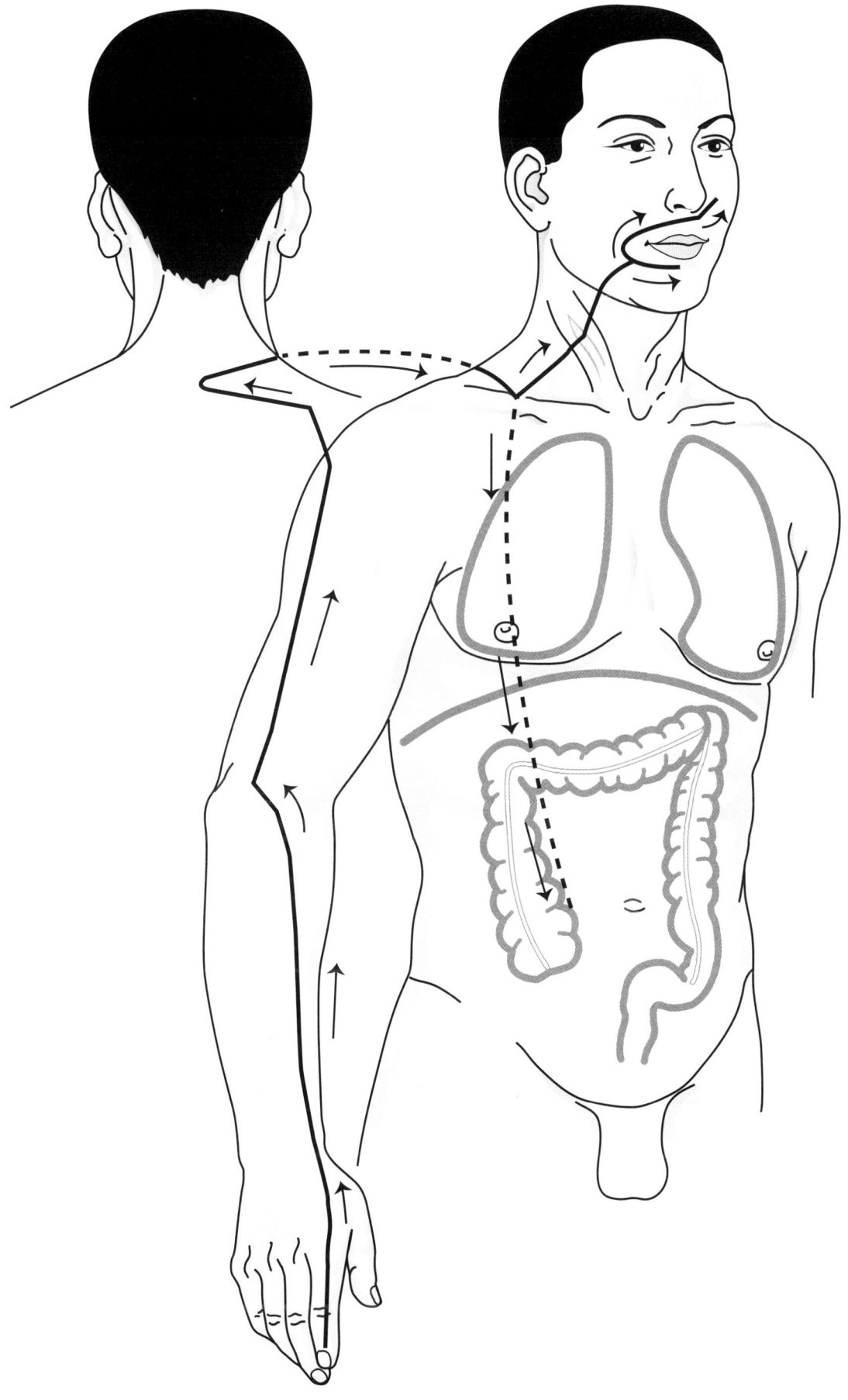

Figure 2.2 Large Intestine Channel — Stage 2

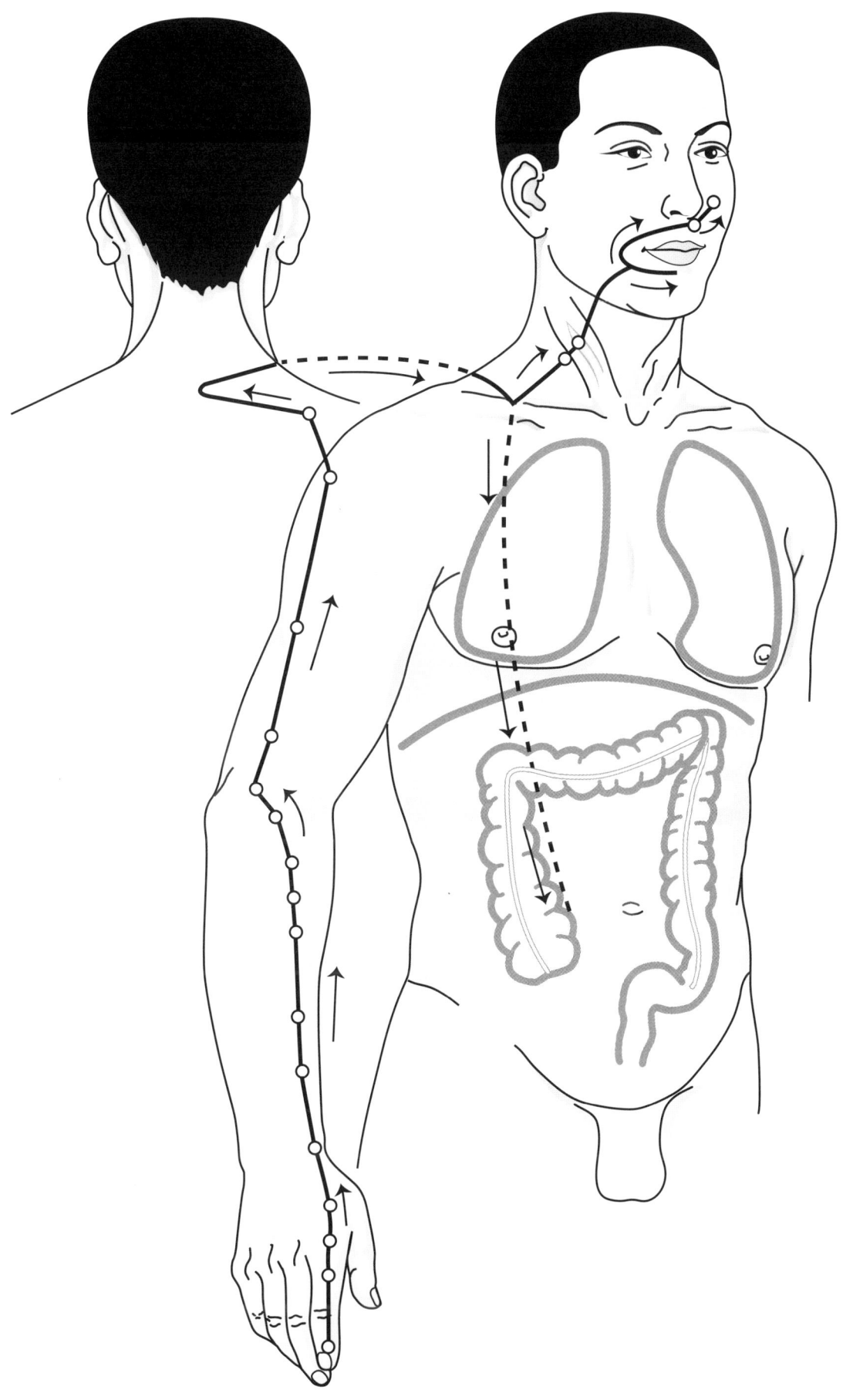

Figure 2.3 Large Intestine Channel — Stage 3

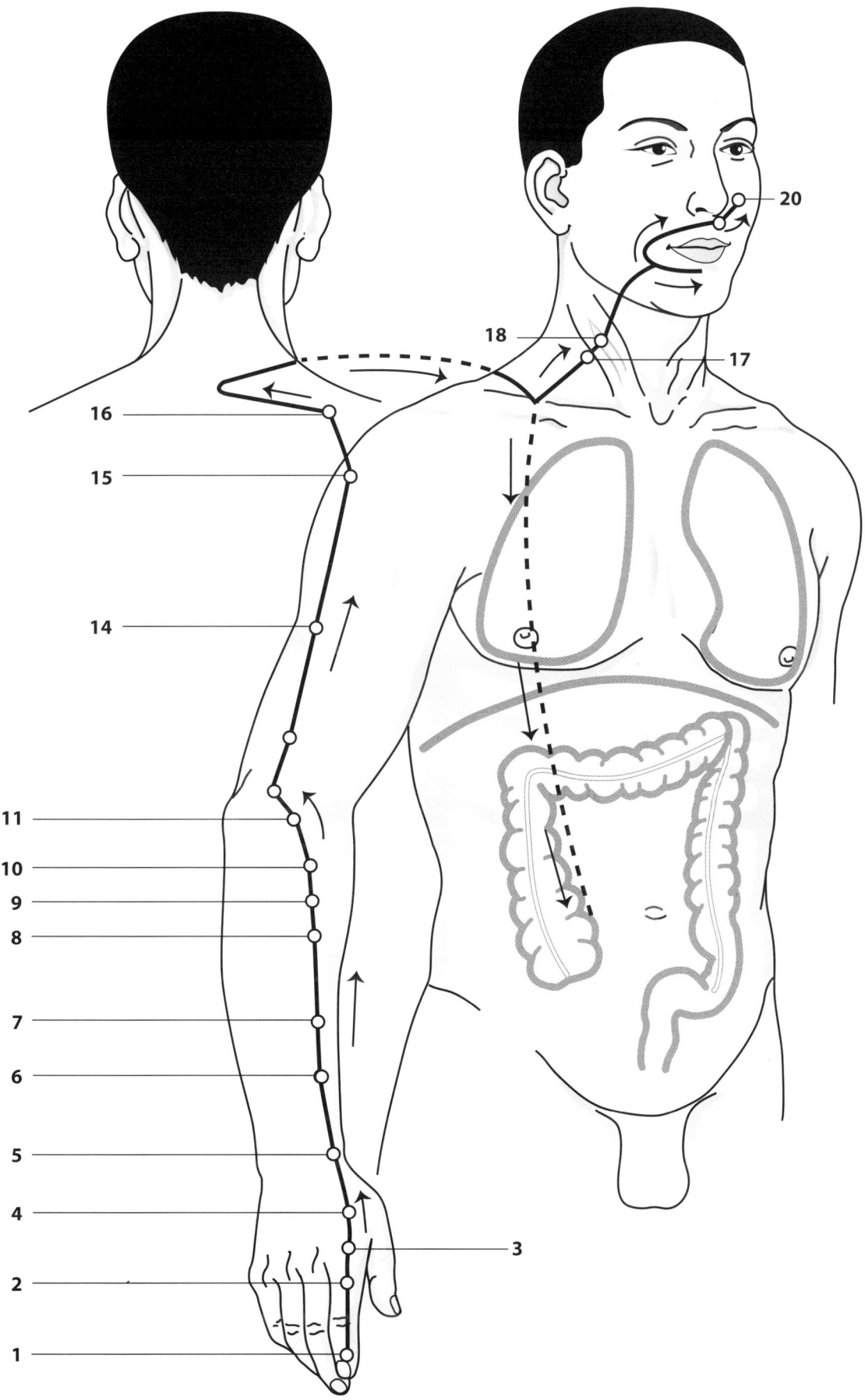

Figure 2.4 Large Intestine Channel — Stage 4

yuan — blue
luo — red
xi-cleft — green
five shu — yellow
lower he-sea — orange
back-shu — purple

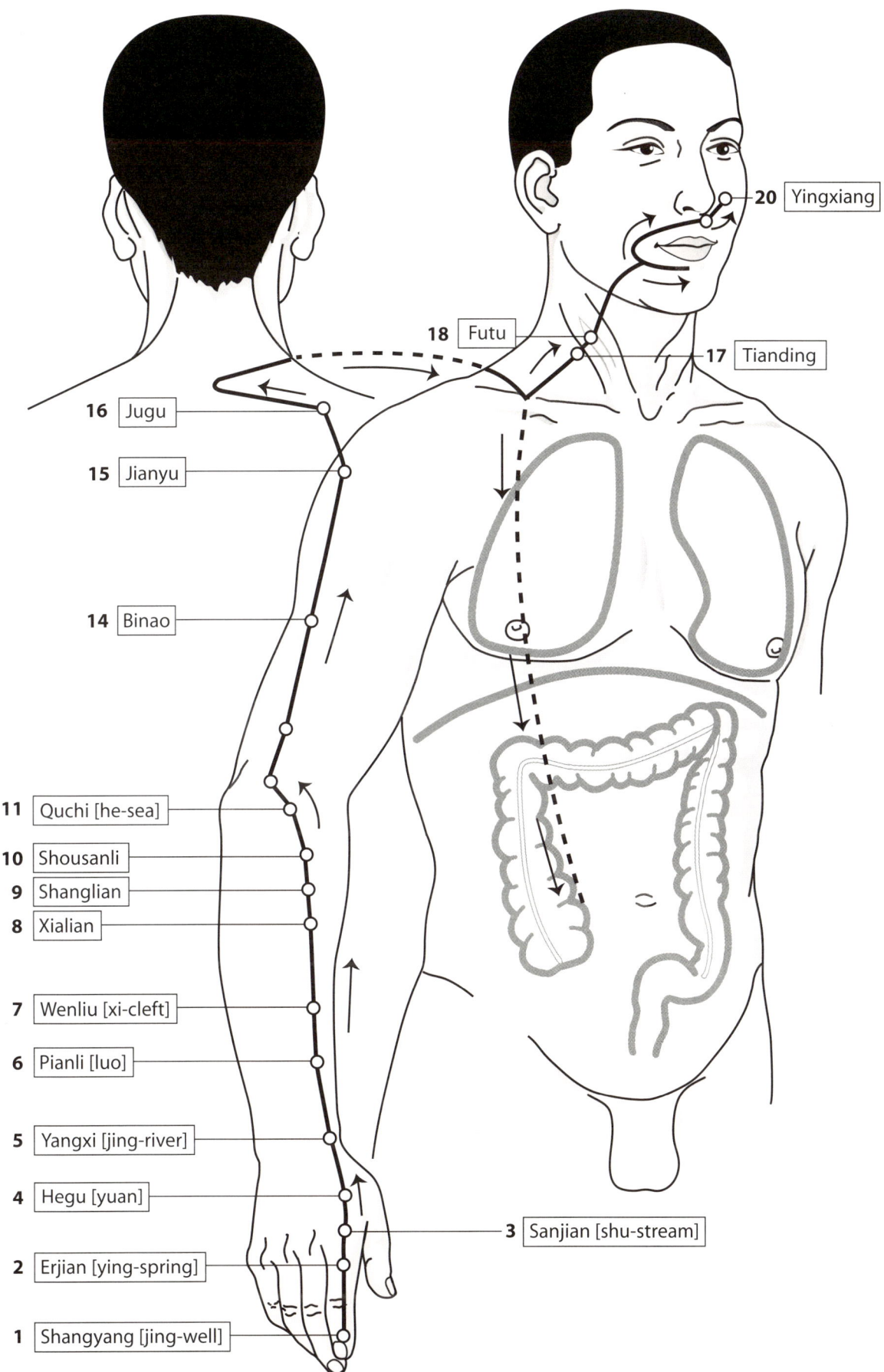

20 Yingxiang

18 Futu

17 Tianding

16 Jugu

15 Jianyu

14 Binao

11 Quchi [he-sea]

10 Shousanli

9 Shanglian

8 Xialian

7 Wenliu [xi-cleft]

6 Pianli [luo]

5 Yangxi [jing-river]

4 Hegu [yuan]

3 Sanjian [shu-stream]

2 Erjian [ying-spring]

1 Shangyang [jing-well]

Figure 2.5 Large Intestine Channel — Stage 5

THE LARGE INTESTINE CHANNEL — CASE STUDY

> ### Mr DC, 24 year old rugby player
>
> Mr DC is injured during a heavy tackle, while playing rugby. He presents with an acutely painful right shoulder. He complains of intense localised stabbing pain (9/10), restricted arm movements, bruising, swelling and slightly warm skin over the top of the shoulder, and soreness on the right side of his neck with minor restriction of his neck joints. Examination reveals a rotator cuff strain as a result of trauma from an external force applied to his right shoulder.

QUESTIONS

Circle or write your answers as required.

1 Is this an external or internal disorder?

2 If external:
   (a) Is it due to heat or cold?

   (b) Are there symptoms of wind, dampness or dryness?

   (c) Is it acute, chronic or a mixed condition?

3 If internal:
   (a) Is it due to deficiency or excess?

      (i) If deficient, is it: qi, blood, jin ye, yin or yang?

      (ii) If excess, is it: stagnant qi, stagnant blood, damp/phlegm, rebellious qi, rising liver yang, empty fire etc?

   (b) Is it due to cold or heat?

   (c) Which zang fu are affected?

   (d) Which channels are affected?

4 What might the pulse feel like?
   Describe: pulse rate, rhythm, depth, shape and strength.

5 What might the tongue look like?
   Describe:
   – tongue body (colour, shape, thickness)
   – tongue coating (moisture, colour, thickness, distribution, root).

6 What is the Chinese diagnosis?
   Where appropriate discuss the root (ben), the presenting symptoms (biao) and the five phase/ wu xing dynamics (the relationship between and among the zang fu organs under syndromes of imbalance or disease).

7 What is your treatment principle?

8 What points would you use and why? Include adjunctive therapy such as moxa or cupping, if appropriate.
   (A minimum of five points, use only points on the Lung and Large Intestine Channels.)

Chapter Three

THE STOMACH CHANNEL OF FOOT YANGMING

足太阴脾经

The Stomach Channel of Foot Yangming is *biao li* partnered with the Spleen Channel and paired with the Large Intestine Channel according to six channel theory.

The use of the Stomach Channel is based on knowing the functions and indications of the Stomach Channel points and the pathophysiology of the stomach as a *fu*.

The Stomach Channel connects with the following zang fu:

Stomach   Spleen

The main pathway:

- begins at the lateral side of the nose at Yingxiang LI20, ascending to the medial canthus where it meets the Bladder Channel

- runs along the infra-orbital ridge to Chengqi ST1, descends to enter the upper gum and crosses to join Du Mai at the philtrum

- re-emerges and curves back around the lips to meet Ren Mai in the mento-labial groove

- runs laterally along the jaw line to the angle of the mandible

- ascends in front of the ear, and continues up within the hairline to Touwei ST8 at the forehead where a short branch connects with Du Mai

- the facial branch emerges at Daying ST5, runs down the anterior border of the sternocleidomastoid muscle and enters the supraclavicular fossa where it branches (see other branches below)

- continues downward from the supraclavicular fossa along the mammary line, 4 cun lateral to the midline, as far as Rugen ST18

- continues descending 2 cun lateral to the midline, passing the umbilicus and entering along the lateral side of the inguinal region where it meets another branch descending from the stomach (see other branches below)

- runs down the antero-lateral aspect of the thigh to the knee and from there continues down the antero-lateral aspect of the tibia to the dorsum of the foot

- ends at the lateral side of the tip of the second toe at Lidui ST45.

The other branches:

- the facial branch begins in front of Daying ST5, runs downward along the throat to enter the supraclavicular fossa, travels posteriorly to the upper back to meet Du Mai, descends through the diaphragm, enters the stomach and connects with the spleen

- another branch rises from the pyloric orifice of the stomach, descends inside the abdomen and rejoins the main pathway of the channel at Qichong ST30

- the tibial branch separates from the main pathway at Zusanli ST36 and runs down the lateral margin of the tibia to the lateral side of the middle toe

- a further branch separates on the dorsum of the foot and runs to the medial side of the tip of the big toe, where it links with the Spleen Channel of Foot Taiyin at Yinbai SP1.

The Stomach Channel connects with other primary channels at various points on the body, specifically the Large Intestine, Gall Bladder, Du Mai and Ren Mai Channels.

THE STOMACH CHANNEL POINTS			
WHO number	Pinyin	Name	Specific functions
ST1	**Chengqi**	Tear Container	
ST2	**Sibai**	Four Whites	
ST3	**Juliao**	Great Bone-Hole	
ST4	**Dicang**	Earth Granary	
ST5	**Daying**	Great Reception	
ST6	**Jiache**	Jaw Bone	
ST7	**Xiaguan**	Below the Joint	
ST8	**Touwei**	Head Corner	
ST9	**Renying**	Man's Prognosis	
ST10	Shuitu	Water Prominence	
ST11	Qishe	Qi Abode	
ST12	**Quepen**	Empty Basin	
ST13	**Qihu**	Qi Door	
ST14	Kufang	Store Room	
ST15	Wuyi	Roof	
ST16	Yingchuang	Breast Window	
ST17	**Ruzhong**	Breast Centre	
ST18	**Rugen**	Breast Root	
ST19	**Burong**	Not Contained	
ST20	**Chengman**	Assuming Fullness	
ST21	**Liangmen**	Beam Gate	
ST22	Guanmen	Pass Gate	
ST23	Taiyi	Supreme Unity	
ST24	Huaroumen	Slippery Flesh Gate	
ST25	**Tianshu**	Celestial Pivot	Front-Mu (LI)
ST26	**Wailing**	Outer Mound	
ST27	**Daju**	Great Gigantic	

THE STOMACH CHANNEL POINTS

ST28	**Shuidao**	Waterway	
ST29	**Guilai**	Return	
ST30	**Qichong**	Surging	
ST31	**Biguan**	Thigh Joint	
ST32	**Futu**	Crouching Rabbit	
ST33	Yinshi	Yin Market	
ST34	**Liangqiu**	Beam Hill	Xi-Cleft
ST35	**Dubi**	Calf's Nose	
ST36	**Zusanli**	Leg Three Li	He-Sea*5
ST37	**Shangjuxu**	Upper Great Hollow	Lower He-Sea (LI)
ST38	**Tiaokou**	Ribbon Opening	
ST39	**Xiajuxu**	Lower Great Hollow	Lower He-Sea (SI)
ST40	**Fenglong**	Bountiful Bulge	Luo-Connecting
ST41	**Jiexi**	Ravine Divide	Jing-River*4
ST42	**Chongyang**	Surging Yang	Yuan-Source
ST43	**Xiangu**	Sunken Valley	Shu-Stream*3
ST44	**Neiting**	Inner Court	Ying-Spring*2
ST45	**Lidui**	Severe Mouth	Jing-Well*1

* The 5 Shu points of the Yang Channels:
    1 = metal
    2 = water
    3 = wood
    4 = fire
    5 = earth

Note: The 36 points highlighted in bold are provided on the composite diagram for this channel (the fifth diagram).

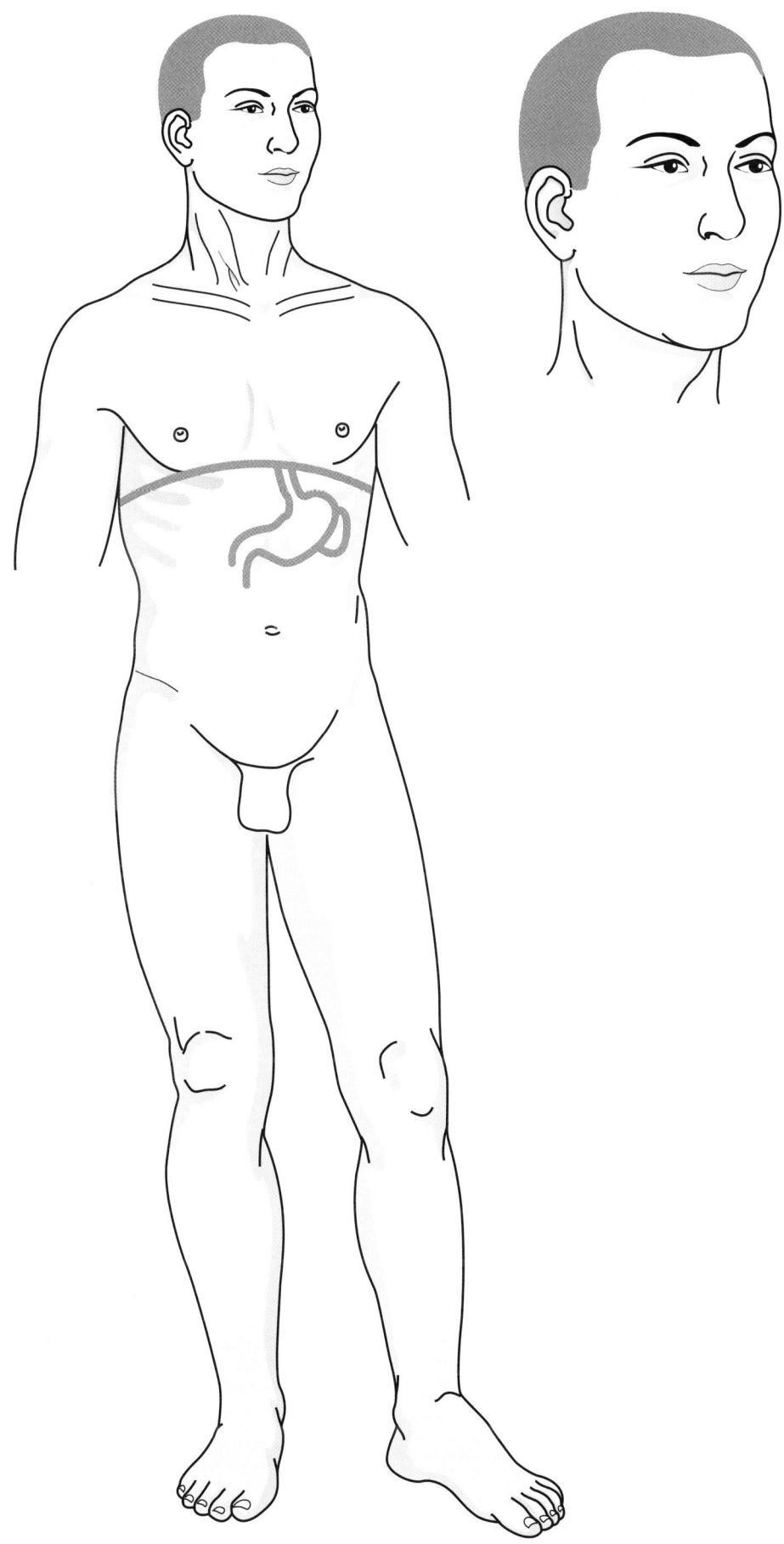

Figure 3.1 Stomach Channel — Stage 1

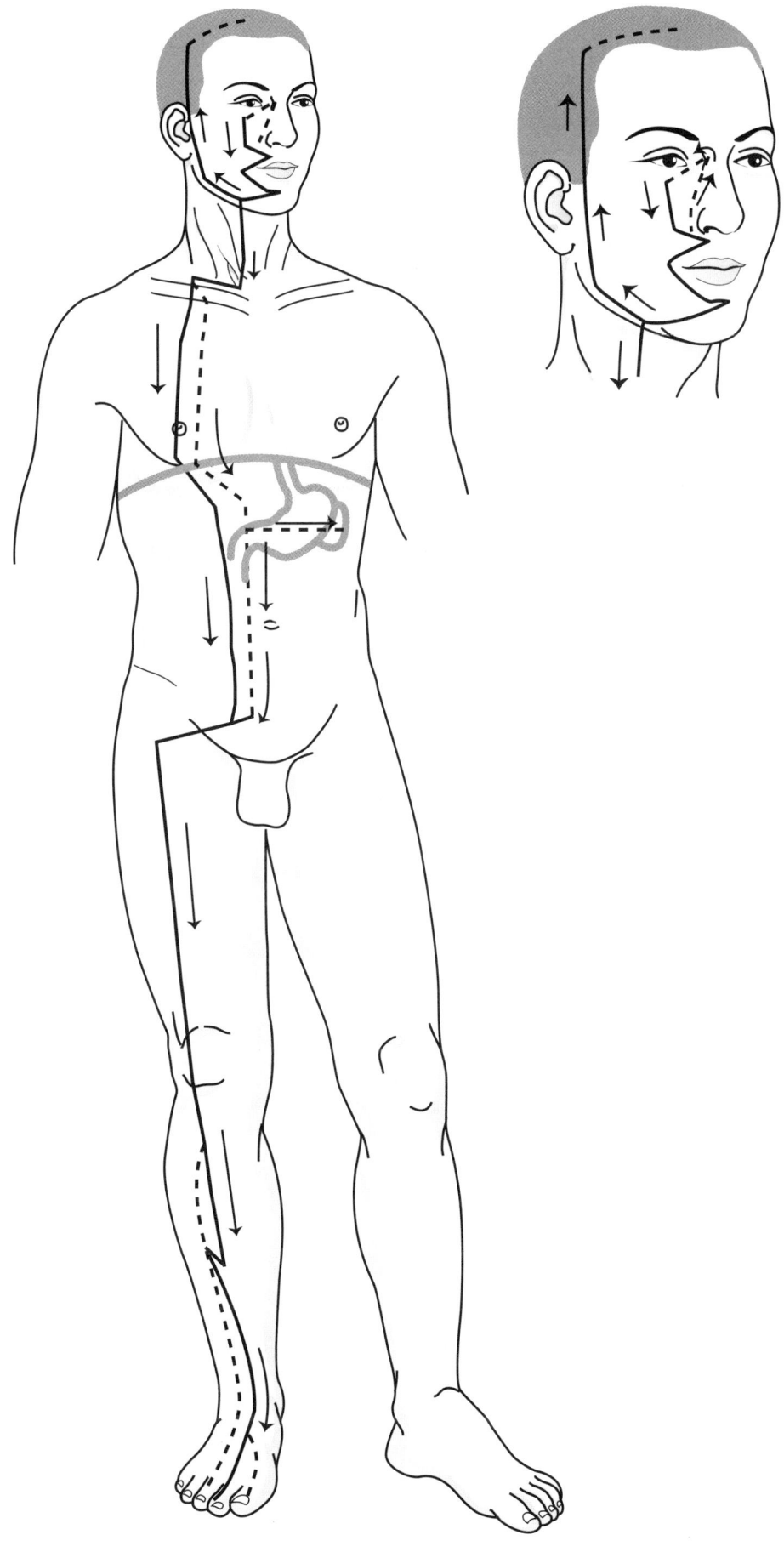

Figure 3.2 Stomach Channel — Stage 2

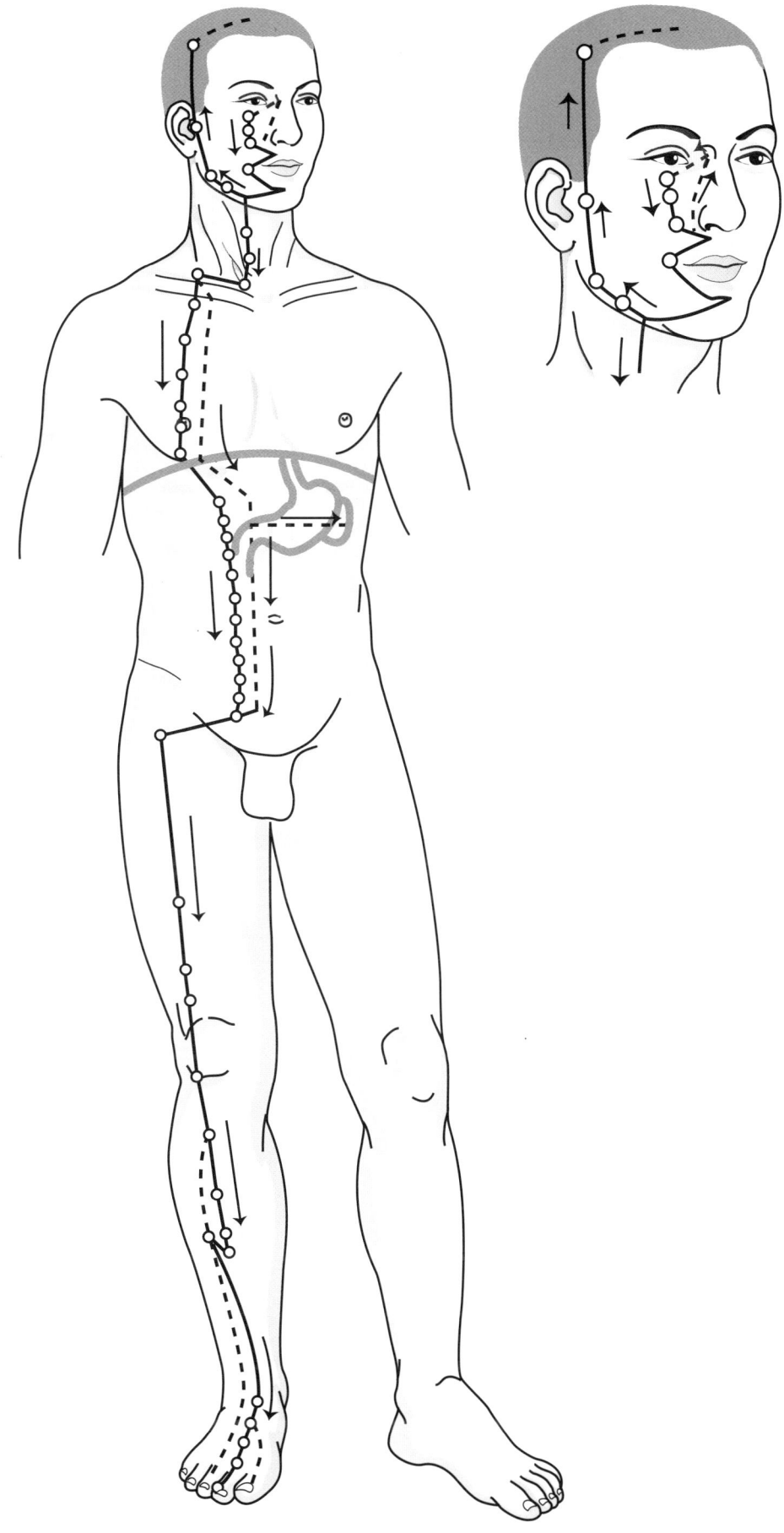

Figure 3.3 Stomach Channel — Stage 3

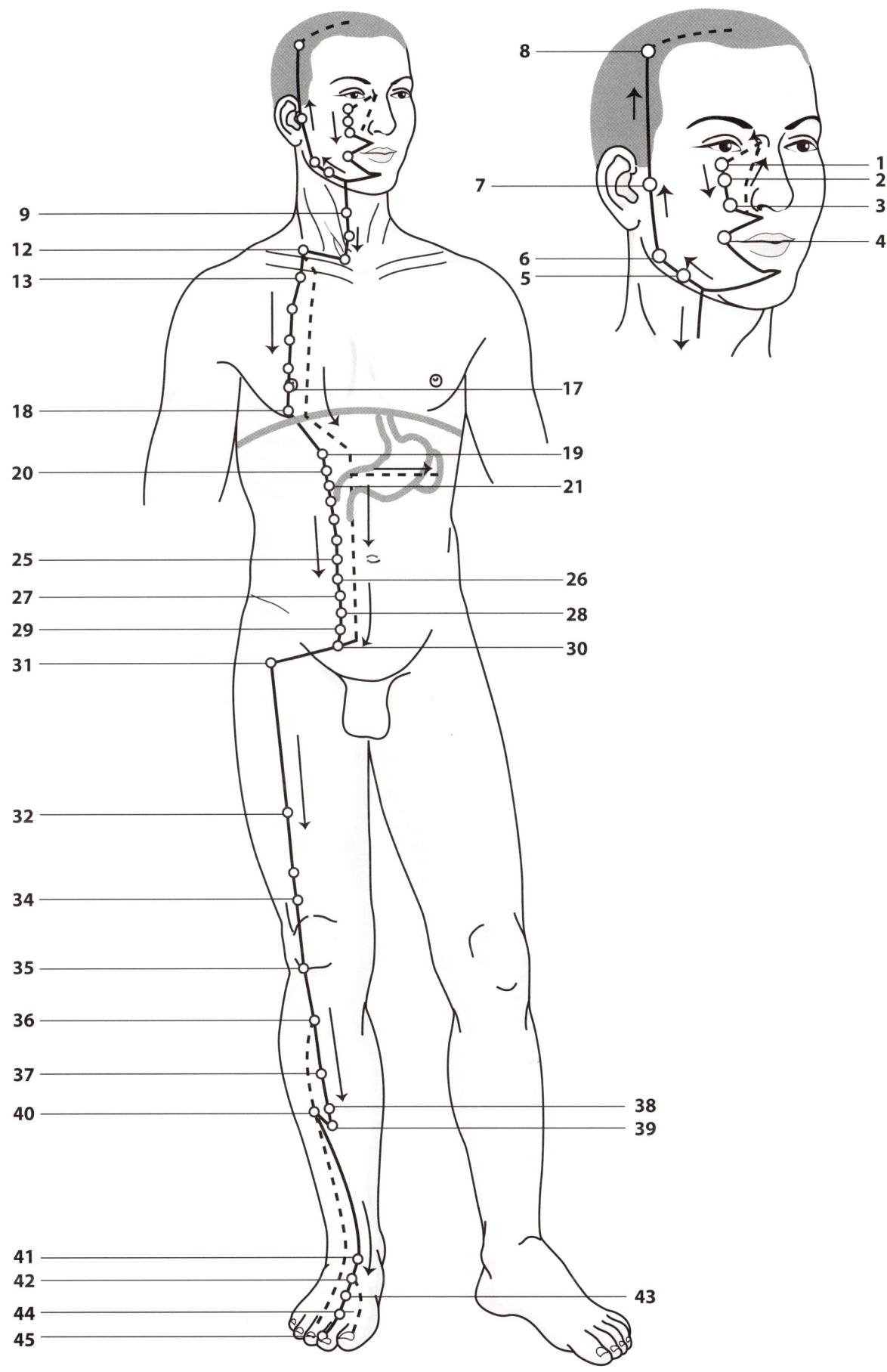

Figure 3.4 Stomach Channel — Stage 4

yuan — blue	
luo — red	
xi-cleft — green	
five shu — yellow	
lower he-sea — orange	
back-shu — purple	

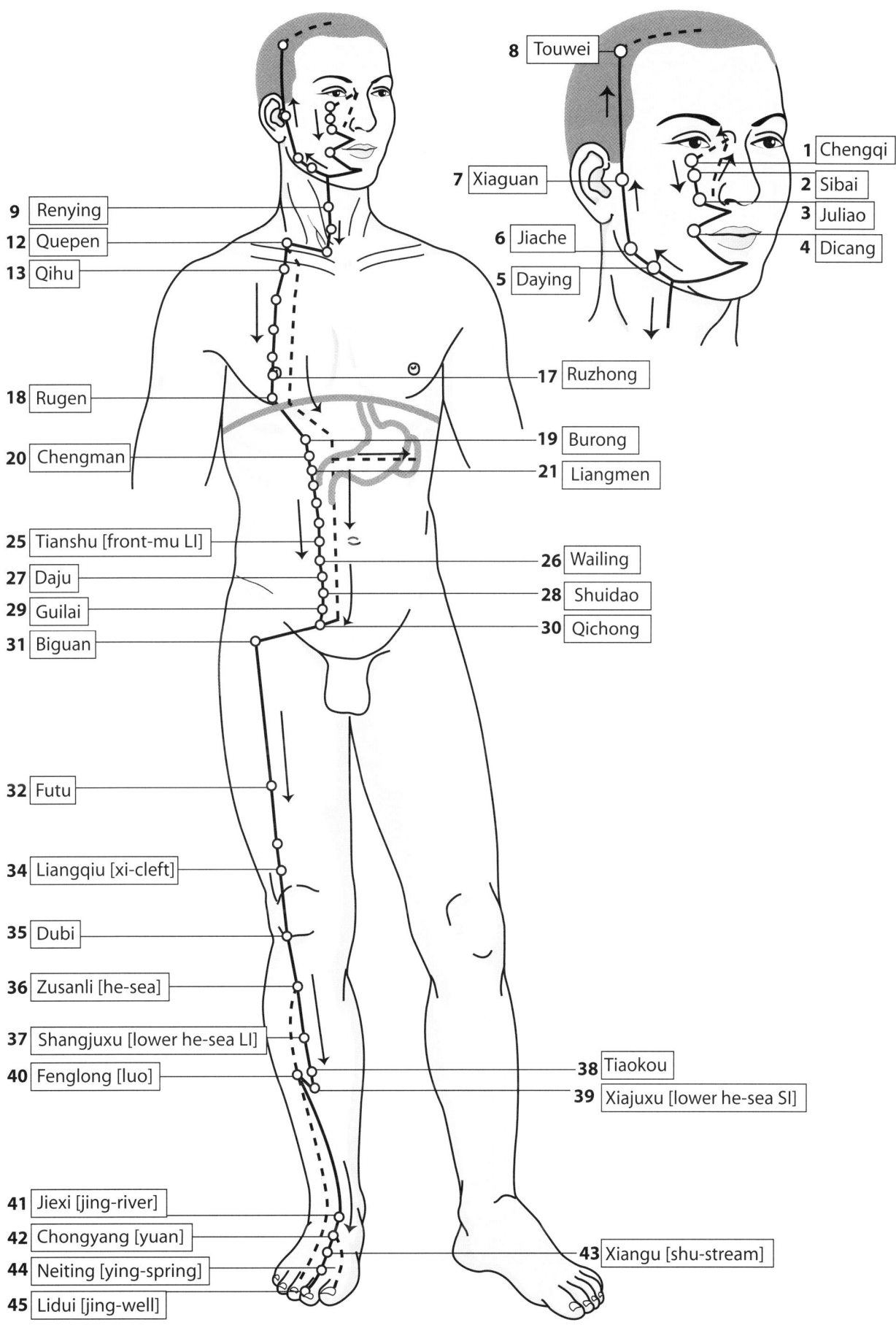

8 Touwei

7 Xiaguan

6 Jiache

5 Daying

1 Chengqi

2 Sibai

3 Juliao

4 Dicang

9 Renying

12 Quepen

13 Qihu

18 Rugen

20 Chengman

25 Tianshu [front-mu LI]

27 Daju

29 Guilai

31 Biguan

32 Futu

34 Liangqiu [xi-cleft]

35 Dubi

36 Zusanli [he-sea]

37 Shangjuxu [lower he-sea LI]

40 Fenglong [luo]

41 Jiexi [jing-river]

42 Chongyang [yuan]

44 Neiting [ying-spring]

45 Lidui [jing-well]

17 Ruzhong

19 Burong

21 Liangmen

26 Wailing

28 Shuidao

30 Qichong

38 Tiaokou

39 Xiajuxu [lower he-sea SI]

43 Xiangu [shu-stream]

Figure 3.5 Stomach Channel — Stage 5

THE STOMACH CHANNEL — CASE STUDY

> **Mr NL, 65 year old retired accountant**
>
> Mr NL presents with a 1 month history of 'stomach upset'. He complains of a lack of appetite, intermittent nausea, feeling thirsty, intermittent acid reflux, belching and some regurgitation of undigested food. He also experiences a sense of fullness 6–8 hours after eating, sharp epigastric pain (8/10) following overeating, spicy foods or eating too quickly, constipation and insomnia (waking in the early hours of the morning).

QUESTIONS

Circle or write your answers as required.

1 Is this an external or internal disorder?

2 If external:

(a) Is it due to heat or cold?

(b) Are there symptoms of wind, dampness or dryness?

(c) Is it acute, chronic or a mixed condition?

3 If internal:

(a) Is it due to deficiency or excess?

   (i)   If deficient, is it: qi, blood, jin ye, yin or yang?

   (ii) If excess, is it: stagnant qi, stagnant blood, damp/phlegm, rebellious qi, rising liver yang, empty fire etc?

(b) Is it due to cold or heat?

(c) Which zang fu are affected?

(d) Which channels are affected?

4 What might the pulse feel like?
Describe: pulse rate, rhythm, depth, shape and strength.

5 What might the tongue look like?
Describe:
- tongue body (colour, shape, thickness)
- tongue coating (moisture, colour, thickness, distribution, root).

6 What is the Chinese diagnosis?
Where appropriate discuss the root (ben), the presenting symptoms (biao) and the five phase/wu xing dynamics (the relationship between and among the zang fu organs under syndromes of imbalance or disease).

7 What is your treatment principle?

8 What points would you use and why? Include adjunctive therapy such as moxa or cupping, if appropriate.
(A minimum of five points, use only points on the Lung, Large Intestine and Stomach Channels.)

Chapter Four

THE SPLEEN CHANNEL OF FOOT TAIYIN

足太阴脾经

The Spleen Channel of Foot Taiyin is *biao li* partnered with the Stomach Channel and paired with the Large Intestine Channel according to six channel theory.

The use of the Spleen Channel is based on knowing the functions and indications of the Spleen Channel points and the pathophysiology of the spleen as a *zang*.

The Spleen Channel connects with the following zang fu:

Spleen   Stomach   Heart

The main pathway:

- begins at the medial side of the big toe at Yinbai SP1 and runs along the medial aspect of the foot at the junction of the pink and white skin

- ascends in front of the medial malleolus and follows the posterior border of the tibia on the medial aspect of the leg

- crosses in front of the Liver Channel of Foot Jueyin

- continues upward through the antero-medial aspect of the knee and thigh

- enters the abdomen, intercepts Ren Mai, enters the spleen and connects with the stomach

- ascends 4 cun lateral to the midline to Fuai SP16, then continues upward 6 cun lateral to the midline until the second intercostal space

- just superior to Zhongfu LU1, it descends to end 6 cun below the axilla in the mid-auxiliary line (sixth or seventh intercostal space) at Dabao SP21.

The other branches:

- the stomach branch pierces the diaphragm, runs upward alongside the oesophagus and when it reaches the root of the tongue, spreads over its lower surface

- another branch begins from the stomach, ascends up through the diaphragm and flows into the heart to link with the Heart Channel of Hand Shaoyin.

The Spleen Channel connects with other primary channels at various points on the body, specifically the Lung, Liver, Gall Bladder and Ren Mai Channels.

WHO number	Pinyin	Name	Specific functions
		THE SPLEEN CHANNEL POINTS	
SP1	**Yinbai**	Hidden White	Jing-Well*1
SP2	**Dadu**	Great Metropolis	Ying-Spring*2
SP3	**Taibai**	Supreme White	Yuan-Source, Shu-Stream*3
SP4	**Gongsun**	Yellow Emperor	Luo-Connecting, Confluent Chong Mai
SP5	**Shangqiu**	Shang Hill	Jing-River*4
SP6	**Sanyinjiao**	Three Yin Intersection	
SP7	**Lougu**	Leaking Valley	
SP8	**Diji**	Earth's Crux	Xi-Cleft
SP9	**Yinlingquan**	Yin Mound Spring	He-Sea*5
SP10	**Xuehai**	Sea of Blood	
SP11	Jimen	Winnower Gate	
SP12	**Chongmen**	Surging Gate	
SP13	Fushe	Bowel Abode	
SP14	Fujie	Abdominal Bind	
SP15	**Daheng**	Great Horizontal	
SP16	**Fuai**	Abdominal Lament	
SP17	Shidou	Food Hole	
SP18	Tianxi	Celestial Ravine	
SP19	Xiongxiang	Chest Village	
SP20	Zhourong	All-Round Flourishing	
SP21	**Dabao**	Great Embracement	Great Luo-Connecting point

* The 5 Shu points of the Yin Channels:

   1 = wood
   2 = fire
   3 = earth
   4 = metal
   5 = water

Note: The 14 points highlighted in bold are provided on the composite diagram for this channel (the fifth diagram).

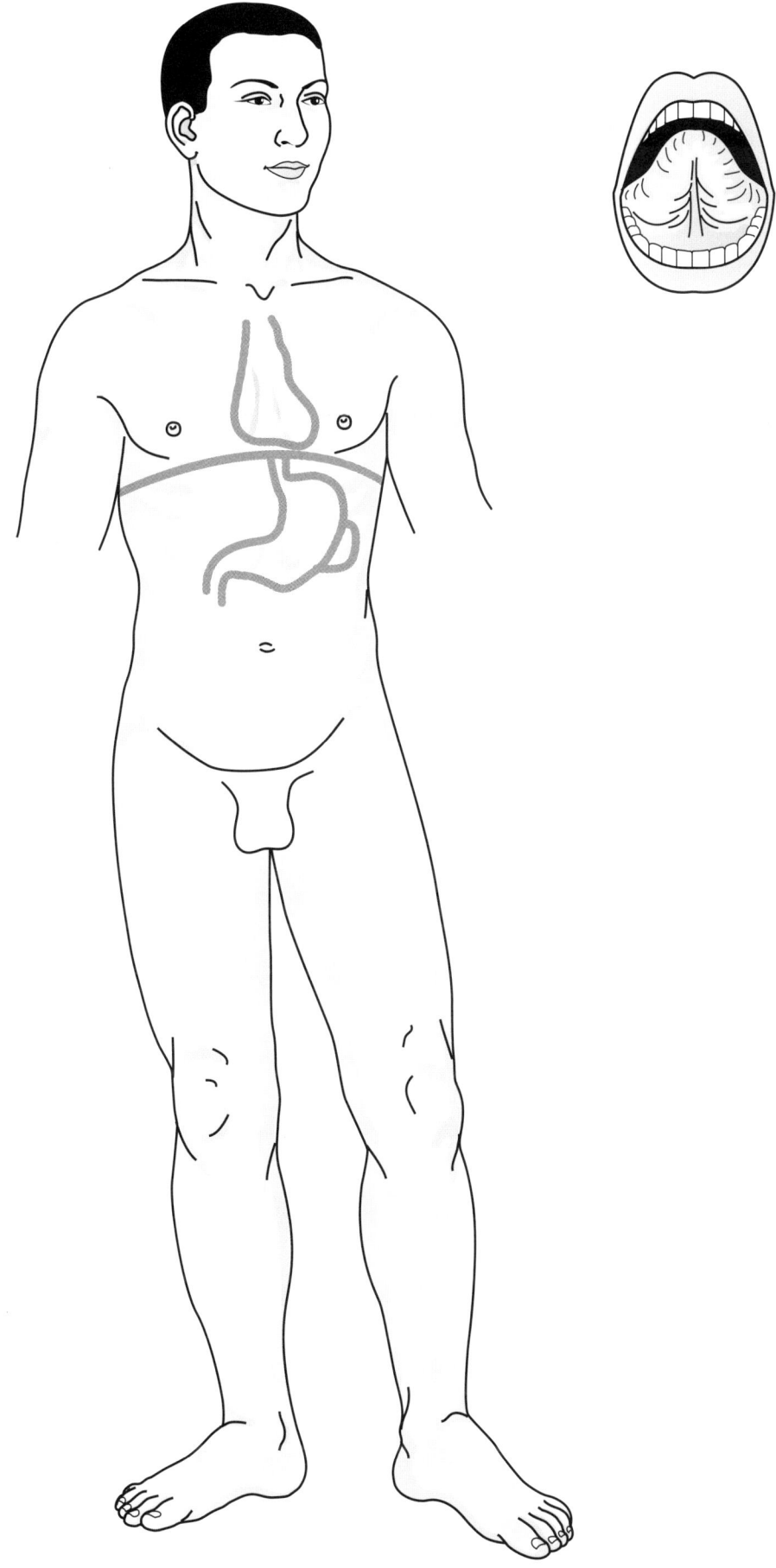

Figure 4.1 Spleen Channel — Stage 1

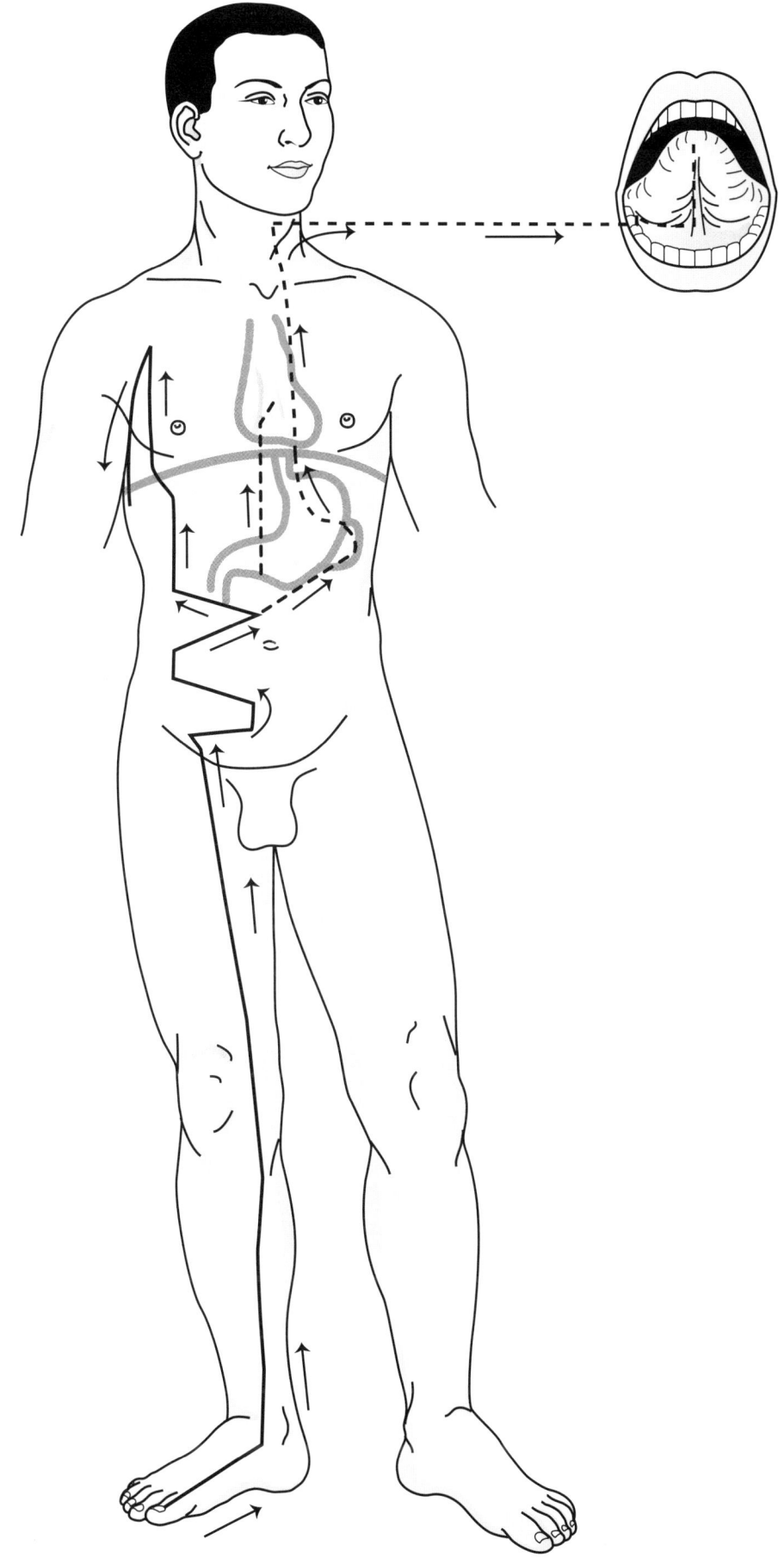

Figure 4.2 Spleen Channel — Stage 2

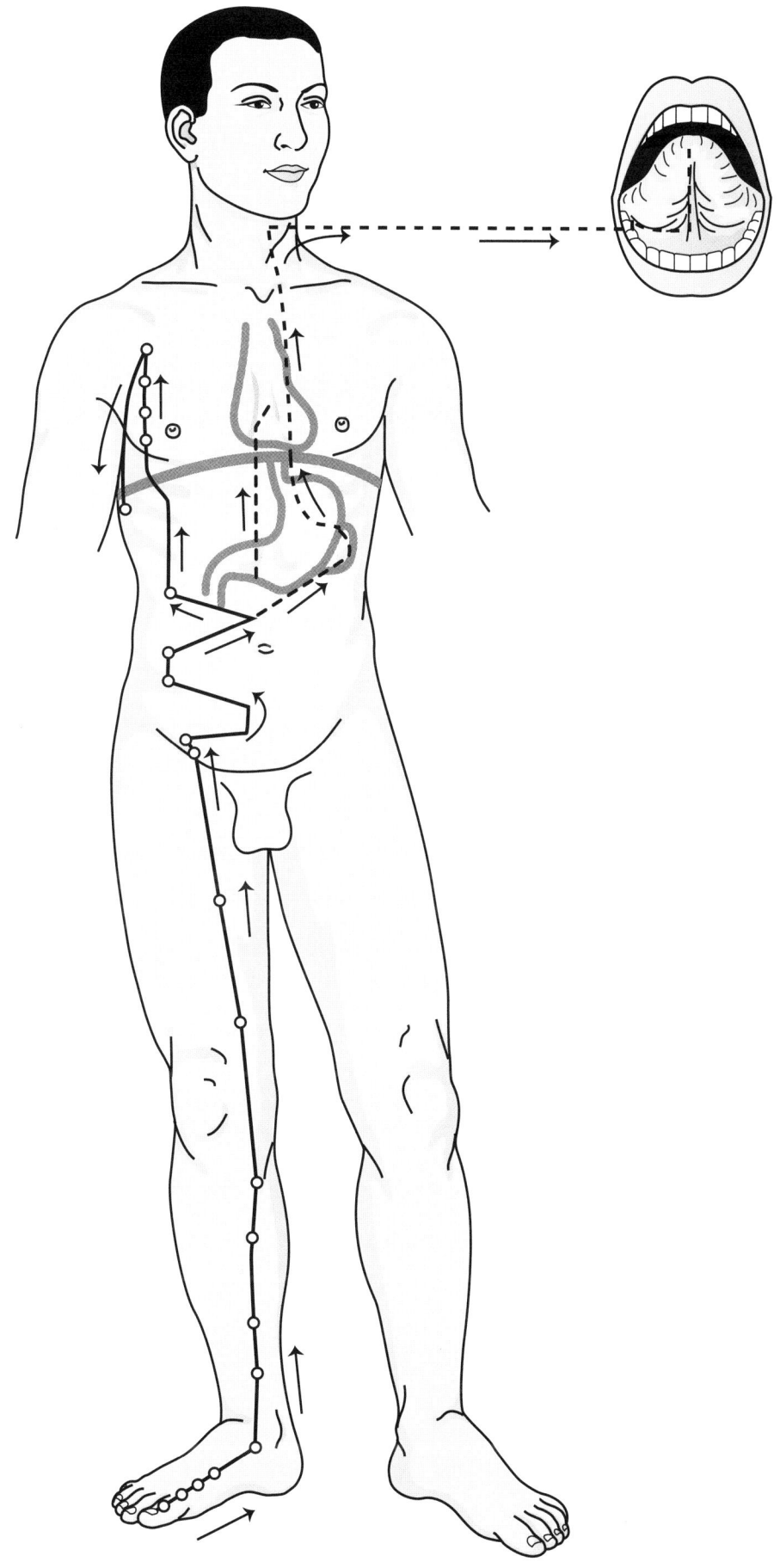

Figure 4.3 Spleen Channel — Stage 3

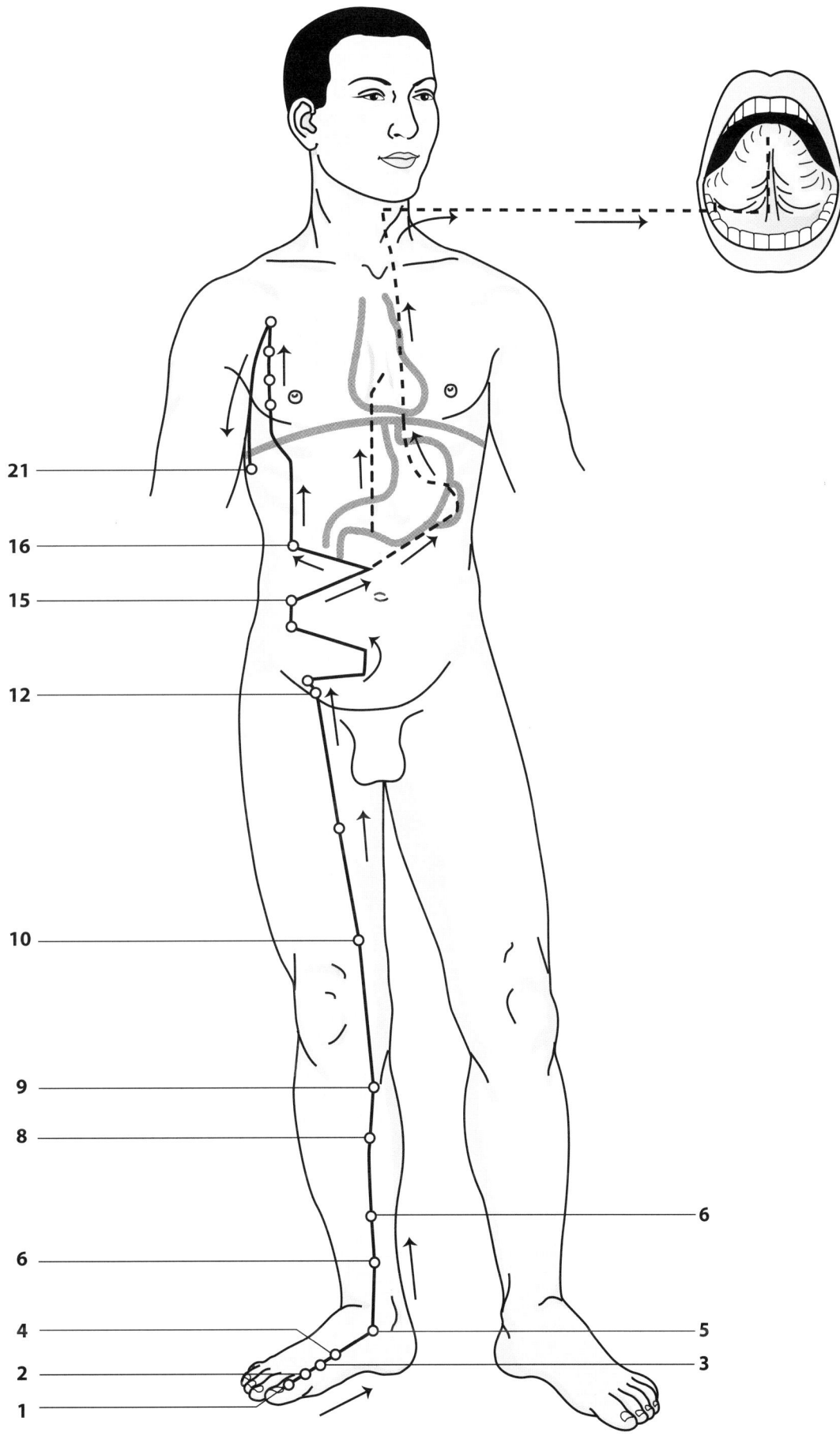

Figure 4.4 Spleen Channel — Stage 4

yuan — blue	
luo — red	
xi-cleft — green	
five shu — yellow	
lower he-sea — orange	
back-shu — purple	

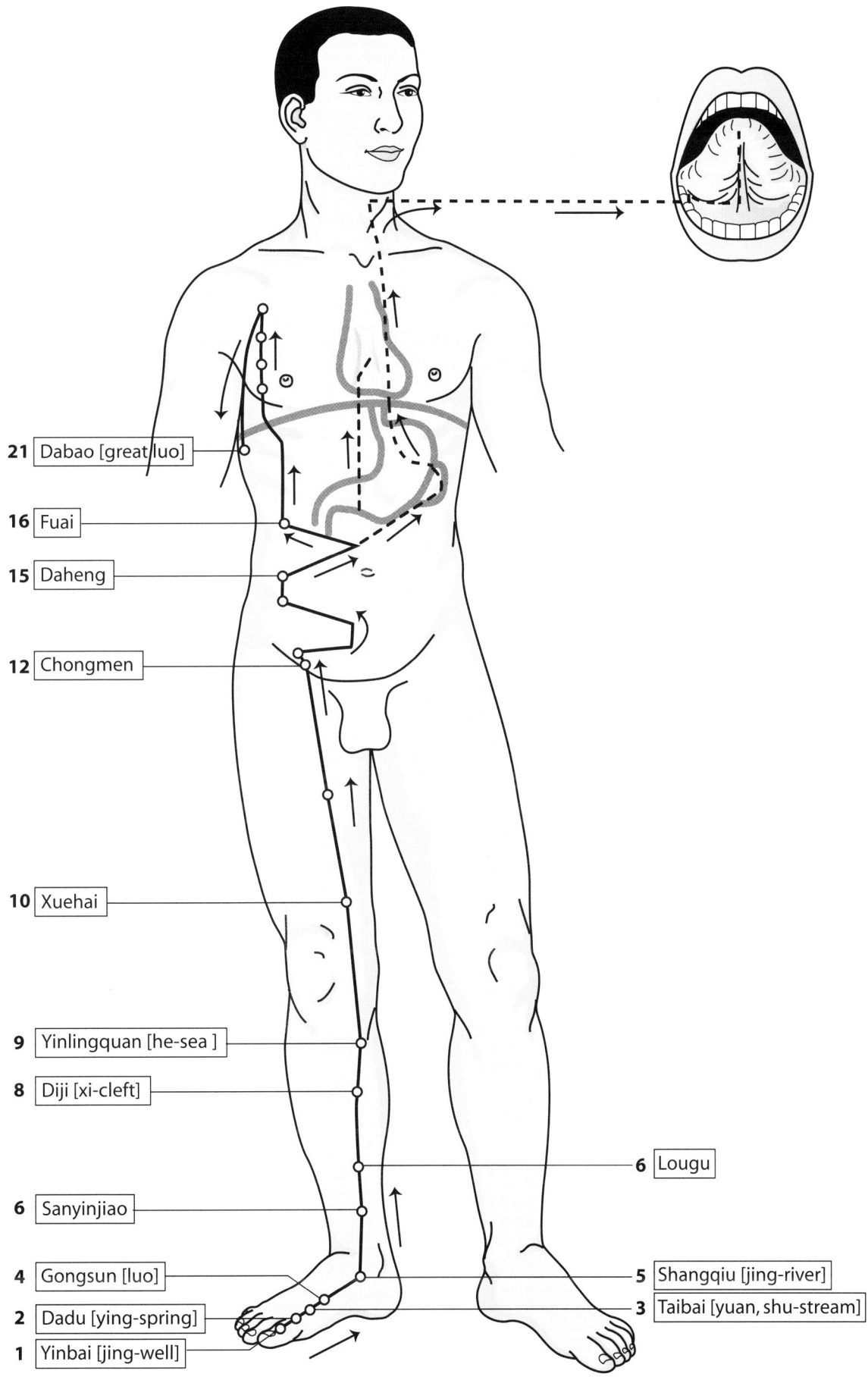

21 Dabao [great luo]

16 Fuai

15 Daheng

12 Chongmen

10 Xuehai

9 Yinlingquan [he-sea]

8 Diji [xi-cleft]

6 Lougu

6 Sanyinjiao

5 Shangqiu [jing-river]

4 Gongsun [luo]

3 Taibai [yuan, shu-stream]

2 Dadu [ying-spring]

1 Yinbai [jing-well]

Figure 4.5 Spleen Channel — Stage 5

THE SPLEEN CHANNEL — CASE STUDY

Ms HT, 36 year old corporate consultant

Ms HT has been feeling stressed and pressured at work for the last few months. She complains of feeling tired, eating on the run, weight gain, a sallow complexion, heaviness and abdominal fullness following food, loose bowel motions (sometimes with undigested food) up to 4 times per day, and heavy, flooding periods. Recently she has been 'feeling fragile' with poor sleep, waking and worrying about work between 3 a.m. and 5 a.m., and nightmares that wake her 1–2 times per week.

QUESTIONS

Circle or write your answers as required.

1 Is this an external or internal disorder?

2 If external:
   (a) Is it due to heat or cold?

   (b) Are there symptoms of wind, dampnes or dryness?

   (c) Is it acute, chronic or a mixed condition?

3 If internal:
   (a) Is it due to deficiency or excess?

      (i) If deficient, is it: qi, blood, jin ye, yin or yang?

      (ii) If excess, is it: stagnant qi, stagnant blood, damp/phlegm, rebellious qi, rising liver yang, empty fire etc?

   (b) Is it due to cold or heat?

   (c) Which zang fu are affected?

   (d) Which channels are affected?

4 What might the pulse feel like?
   Describe: pulse rate, rhythm, depth, shape and strength.

5 What might the tongue look like?
   Describe:
   – tongue body (colour, shape, thickness)
   – tongue coating (moisture, colour, thickness, distribution, root).

6 What is the Chinese diagnosis?
   Where appropriate discuss the root (ben), the presenting symptoms (biao) and the five phase/ wu xing dynamics (the relationship between and among the zang fu organs under syndromes of imbalance or disease).

7 What is your treatment principle?

8 What points would you use and why? Include adjunctive therapy such as moxa or cupping, if appropriate.
   (A minimum of five points, use only points on the Lung, Large Intestine, Stomach and Spleen Channels.)

Chapter Five

THE HEART CHANNEL OF HAND SHAOYIN

手少阴心经

The Heart Channel of Hand Shaoyin is *biao li* partnered with the Small Intestine Channel and paired with the Kidney Channel according to six channel theory.

The use of the Heart Channel is based on knowing the functions and indications of the Heart Channel points and the pathophysiology of the heart as a *zang*.

The Heart Channel connects with the following zang fu:

Heart   Lung   Small Intestine

The main pathway:

- emerges from the axilla at Jiquan HT1

- travels down the ventral aspect of the medial border of the arm, medial to the Pericardium and Lung Channels

- passes through the ante-cubital fossa and descends along the antero-medial aspect of the forearm, on the radial side of the ulna tendon

- at the depression proximal to the pisiform bone it enters the palm and follows the radial aspect of the little finger to its tip, linking with the Small Intestine Channel of Hand Taiyang at Shaochong HT9.

The other branches:

- originate in the heart
- one branch emerges from the system of blood vessels and tissues surrounding the heart and descends through the diaphragm to connect with the small intestine
- a second branch from the heart ascends alongside the oesophagus and up across the cheek to connect with the tissues surrounding the eye
- a third branch arches away from the heart to the lung and descends to emerge from the axilla at Jiquan HT1 (see main pathway above).

The Heart Channel has no connections with other primary channels at any points on the body.

THE HEART CHANNEL POINTS			
WHO number	**Pinyin**	**Name**	**Specific functions**
HT1	**Jiquan**	Higher Spring	
HT2	**Qingling**	Cyan Spirit	
HT3	**Shaohai**	Lesser Sea	He-Sea*1
HT4	**Lingdao**	Spirit Pathway	Jing-River*4
HT5	**Tongli**	Connecting Li	Luo-Connecting
HT6	**Yinxi**	Yin Cleft	Xi-Cleft
HT7	**Shenmen**	Spirit Gate	Yuan-Source, Shu-Stream*3
HT8	**Shaofu**	Lesser Mansion	Ying-Spring*2
HT9	**Shaochong**	Lesser Surge	Jing-Well*1

* The 5 Shu points of the Yin Channels:
    1 = wood
    2 = fire
    3 = earth
    4 = metal
    5 = water

Note: The 9 points highlighted in bold are provided on the composite diagram for this channel (the fifth diagram).

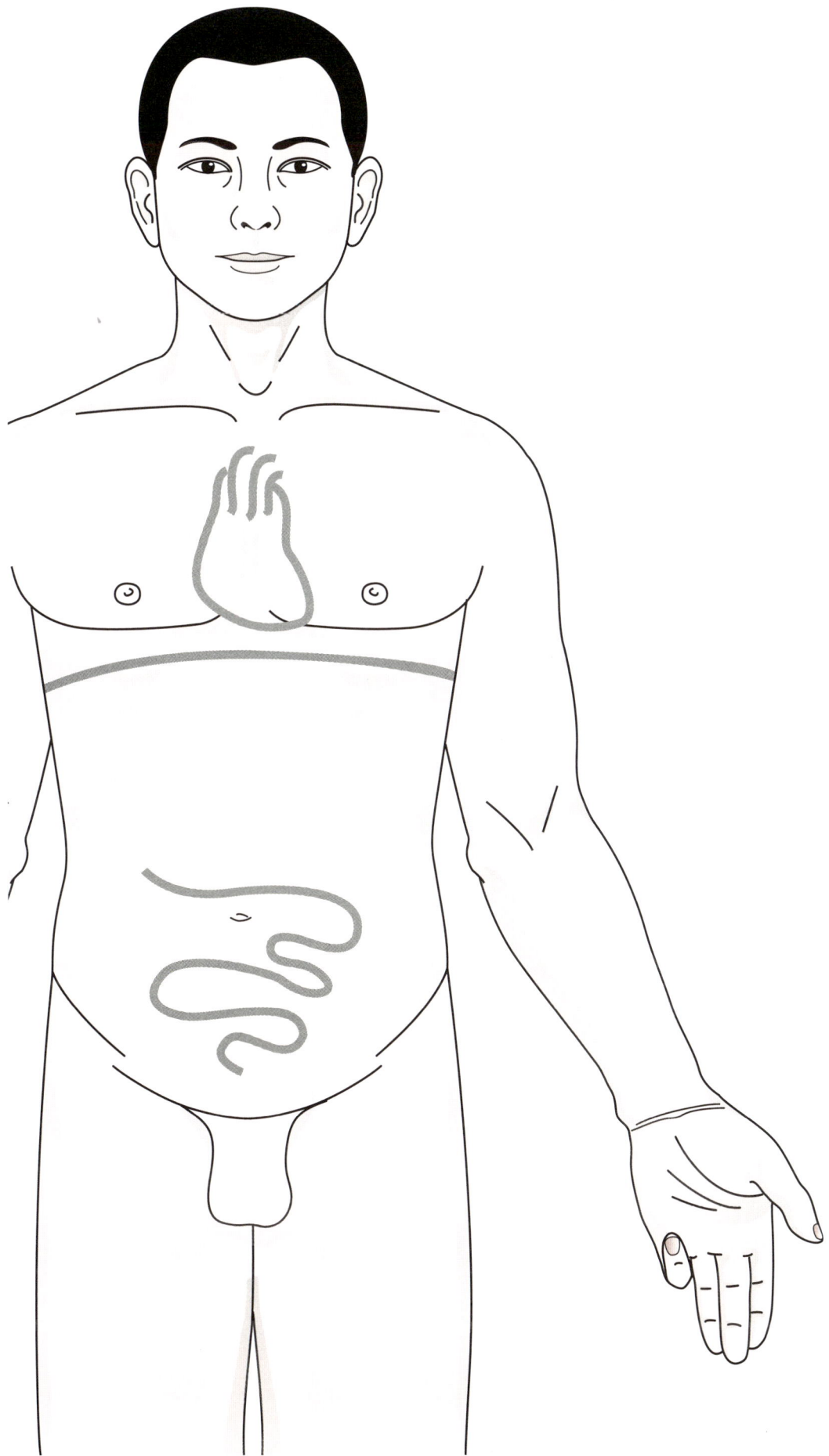

Figure 5.1 Heart Channel — Stage 1

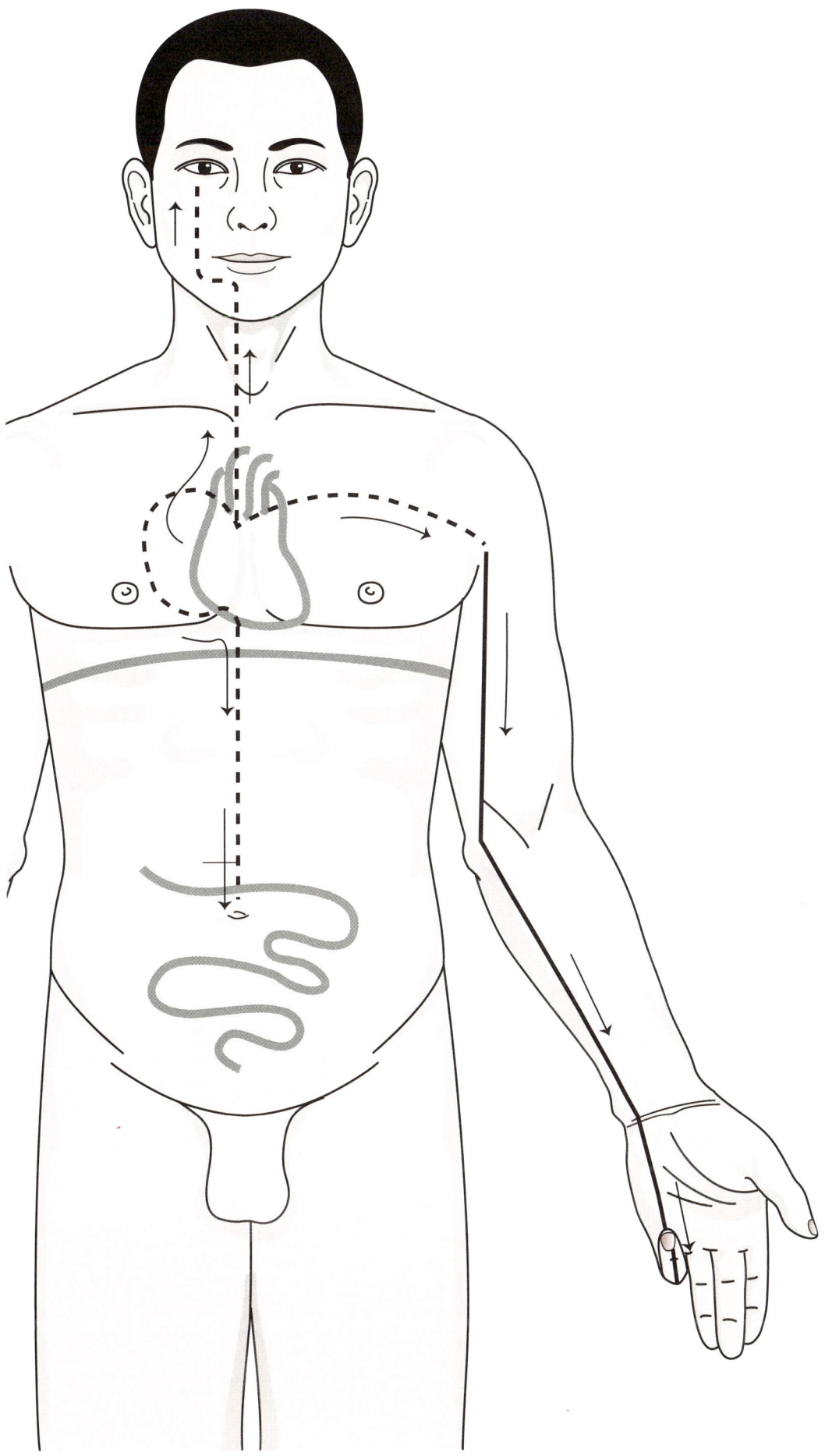

Figure 5.2 Heart Channel — Stage 2

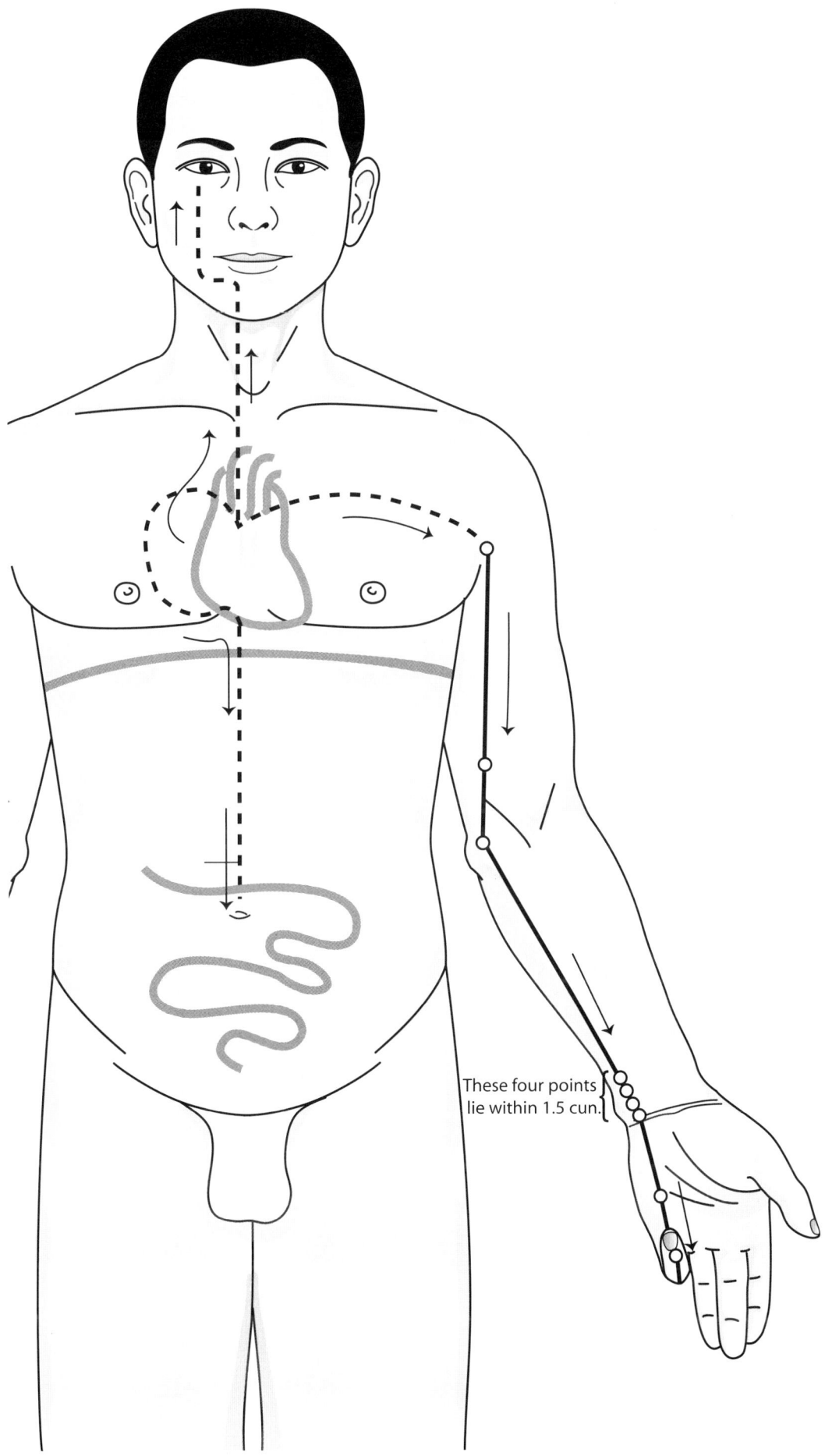

These four points
lie within 1.5 cun.

Figure 5.3 Heart Channel — Stage 3

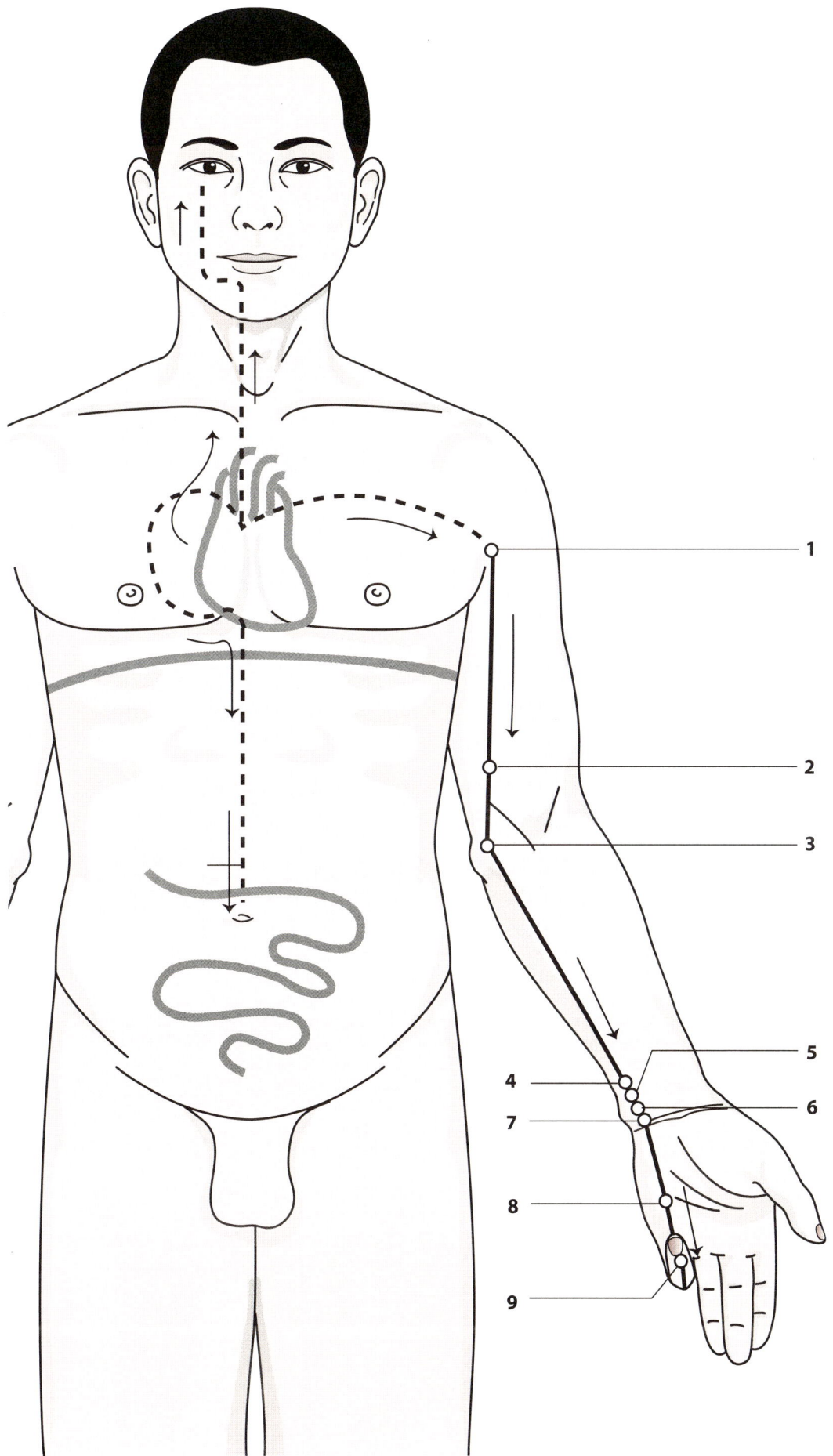

Figure 5.4 Heart Channel — Stage 4

yuan — blue	
luo — red	
xi-cleft — green	
five shu — yellow	
lower he-sea — orange	
back-shu — purple	

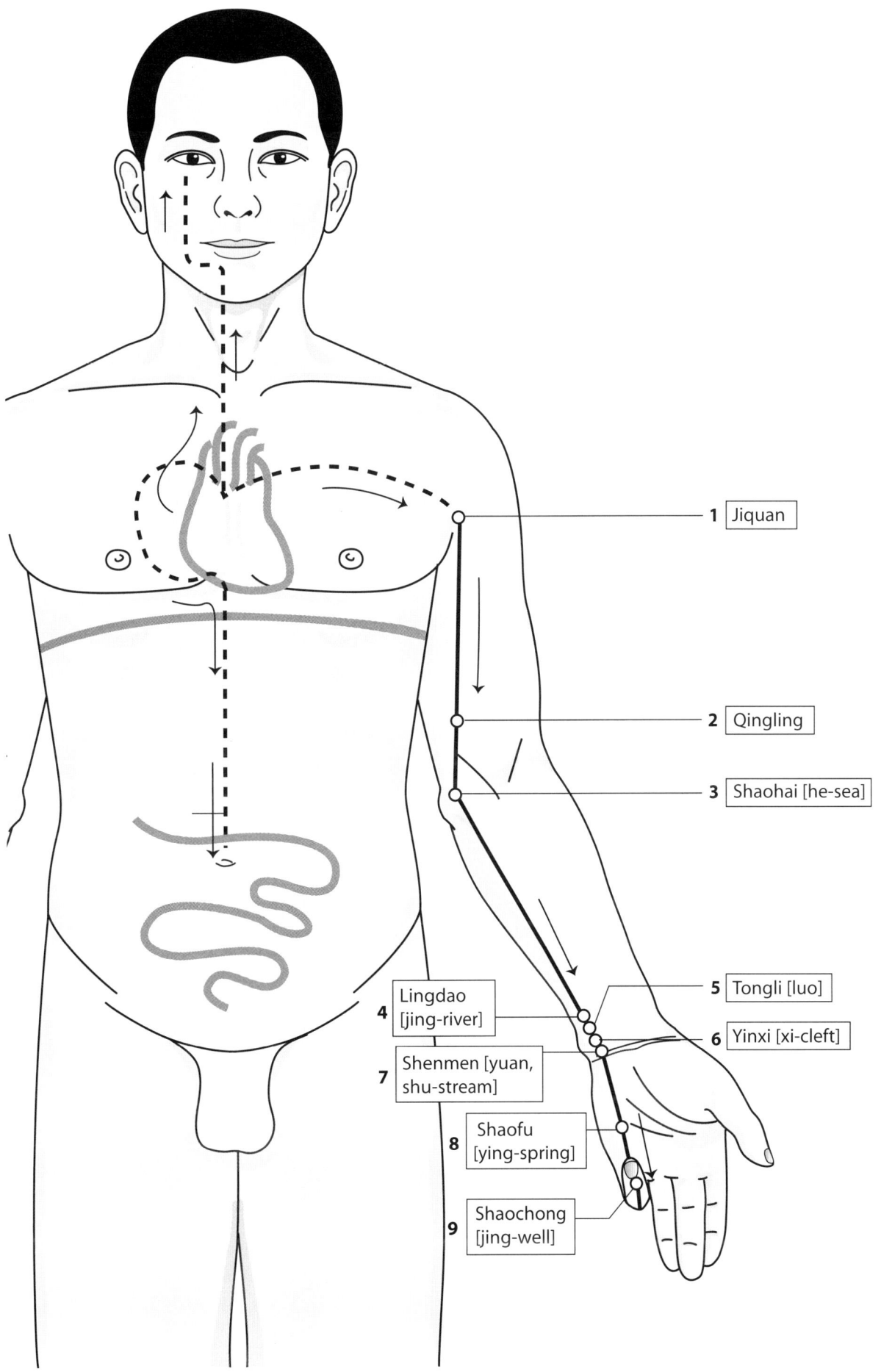

1 Jiquan

2 Qingling

3 Shaohai [he-sea]

5 Tongli [luo]

6 Yinxi [xi-cleft]

4 Lingdao [jing-river]

7 Shenmen [yuan, shu-stream]

8 Shaofu [ying-spring]

9 Shaochong [jing-well]

Figure 5.5 Heart Channel — Stage 5

THE HEART CHANNEL — CASE STUDY

Miss DM, 17 year old schoolgirl preparing for scholarship exams

Miss DM is studying to gain admission to law school. Over the past month she has experienced two to three 'panic attacks' each day. She describes the panic attacks as a feeling of anxiety followed by a sense of panic with shallow fast breathing, a rapid beating heart, tingling around the lips, sweaty palms and upper body, restlessness and wanting to move about or run away. She has difficulty falling asleep at night, and often wakes after midnight feeling hot, sweaty, frightened or 'panic-stricken'. Breathing exercises help.

QUESTIONS

Circle or write your answers as required.

1 Is this an external or internal disorder?

2 If external:

(a) Is it due to heat or cold?

(b) Are there symptoms of wind, dampness or dryness?

(c) Is it acute, chronic or a mixed condition?

3 If internal:

(a) Is it due to deficiency or excess?

(i)   If deficient, is it: qi, blood, jin ye, yin or yang?

(ii) If excess, is it: stagnant qi, stagnant blood, damp/phlegm, rebellious qi, rising liver yang, empty fire etc?

(b) Is it due to cold or heat?

(c) Which zang fu are affected?

(d) Which channels are affected?

4 **What might the pulse feel like?**
   Describe: pulse rate, rhythm, depth, shape and strength.

5 **What might the tongue look like?**
   Describe:
   – tongue body (colour, shape, thickness)
   – tongue coating (moisture, colour, thickness, distribution, root).

6 **What is the Chinese diagnosis?**
   Where appropriate discuss the root (ben), the presenting symptoms (biao) and the five phase/ wu xing dynamics (the relationship between and among the zang fu organs under syndromes of imbalance or disease).

7 **What is your treatment principle?**

8 **What points would you use and why? Include adjunctive therapy such as moxa or cupping, if appropriate.**
   (A minimum of five points, use only points on the Lung, Large Intestine, Stomach, Spleen and Heart Channels.)

Chapter Six

THE SMALL INTESTINE CHANNEL OF HAND TAIYANG

手太阳小肠经

The Small Intestine Channel of Hand Taiyang is *biao li* partnered with the Heart Channel and paired with the Bladder Channel according to six channel theory.

The use of the Small Intestine Channel is based on knowing the functions and indications of the Small Intestine Channel points and the pathophysiology of the small intestine as a *fu*.

The Small Intestine Channel connects with the following zang fu:

Heart   Stomach   Small Intestine

The main pathway:

- begins at the ulnar side of the little finger at Shaoze SI1

- follows the ulnar aspect of the hand to the wrist passing on the radial side of the ulnar styloid

- ascends along the posterior aspect of the forearm to the elbow passing between the olecranon of the ulna and the medial epicondyle of the humerus

- ascends along the posterior aspect of the upper arm to the posterior aspect of the shoulder joint

- then, in a zigzag fashion, descends to the inferior fossa of the scapula and up to the superior fossa of the scapula

- travels to the medial aspect of the scapula spine and upward to the lower border of the spinous process of C7 at Dazhui Du14

- descends into the supraclavicular fossa (see other branches)

- from the supraclavicular fossa, a branch runs up the neck, crosses the cheek to the outer canthus of the eye, and then travels posteriorly towards the ear where it enters the ear at Tinggong SI19

- another branch separates from the neck and runs upward to the infraorbital region at Quanliao SI18, then along the lateral aspect of the nose to the inner canthus of the eye where it meets with the Bladder Channel of Foot Taiyang at Jingming BL1.

The other branches:

- a branch descends from the supraclavicular fossa, runs downward alongside the oesophagus, passes through the heart, diaphragm, stomach and small intestine, intersecting with Ren Mai at three points
- according to the Spiritual Pivot, another branch descends from the small intestine to the lower he-sea point at Xiaojuxu ST39.

The Small Intestine Channel connects with other primary channels at various points on the body, specifically the Large Intestine, Du Mai, Bladder, Stomach, Ren Mai, Gall Bladder and San Jiao Channels.

THE SMALL INTESTINE CHANNEL POINTS			
WHO number	**Pinyin**	**Name**	**Specific functions**
SI1	**Shaoze**	Lesser Marsh	Jing-Well*[1]
SI2	**Qiangu**	Front Valley	Ying-Spring*[2]
SI3	**Houxi**	Back Ravine	Confluent Du Mai, Shu-Stream*[3]
SI4	**Wangu**	Wrist Bone	Yuan-Source
SI5	**Yanggu**	Yang Valley	Jing-River*[4]
SI6	**Yanglao**	Nursing the Aged	Xi-Cleft
SI7	**Zhizheng**	Branch to the Correct	Luo-Connecting
SI8	**Xiaohai**	Small Sea	He-Sea*[5]
SI9	**Jianzhen**	True Shoulder	
SI10	**Naoshu**	Upper Arm Shu	
SI11	**Tianzong**	Celestial Gathering	
SI12	**Bingfeng**	Grasping the Wind	
SI13	**Quyuan**	Crooked Wall	
SI14	**Jianwaishu**	Outer Shoulder Shu	
SI15	**Jianzhongshu**	Central Shoulder Shu	
SI16	**Tianchuang**	Celestial Window	
SI17	**Tianrong**	Celestial Countenance	
SI18	**Quanliao**	Cheek Bone-Hole	
SI19	**Tinggong**	Auditory Palace	

* The 5 Shu points of the Yang Channels:
    1 = metal
    2 = water
    3 = wood
    4 = fire
    5 = earth

Note: The 19 points highlighted in bold are provided on the composite diagram for this channel (the fifth diagram).

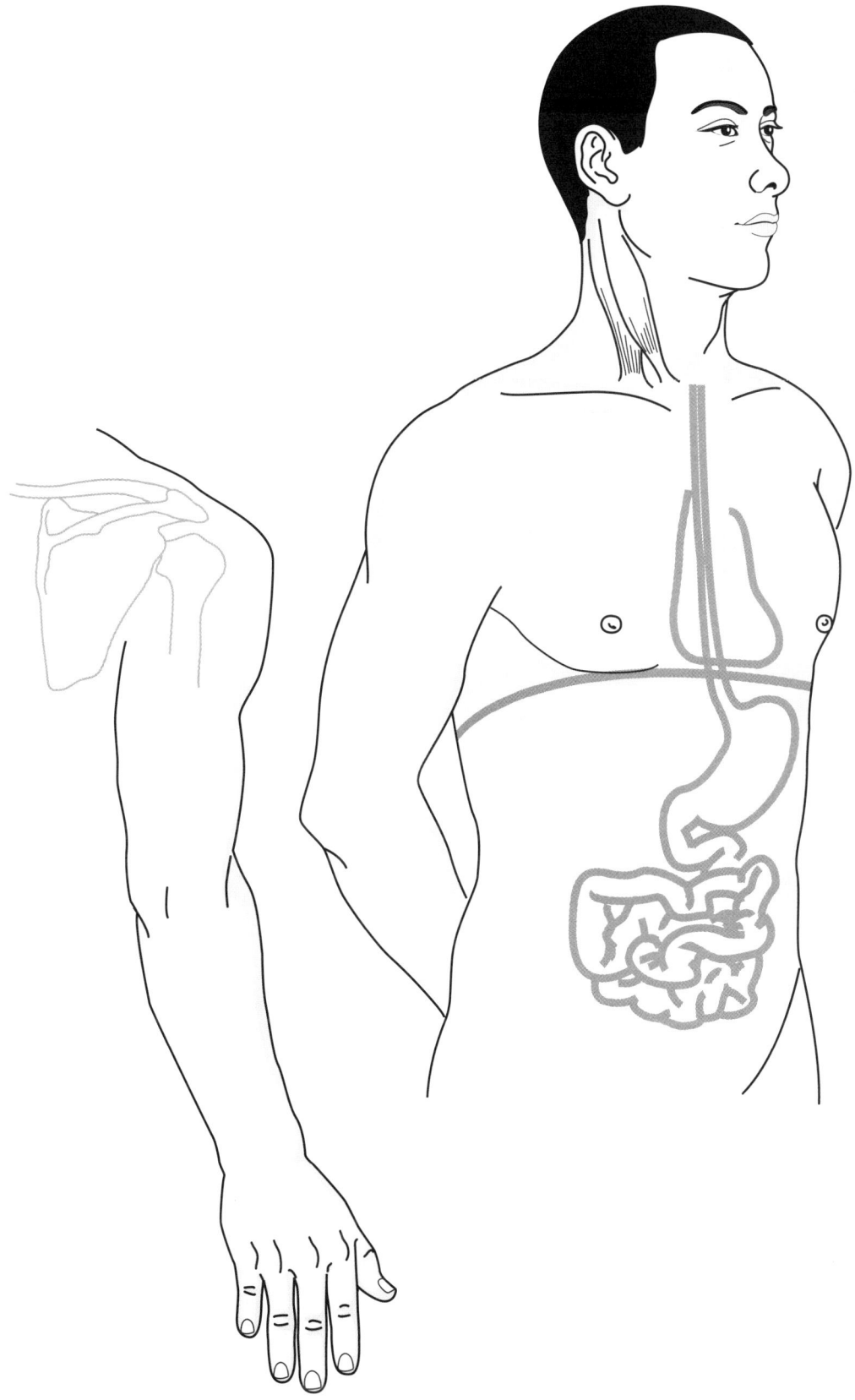

Figure 6.1 Small Intestine Channel — Stage 1

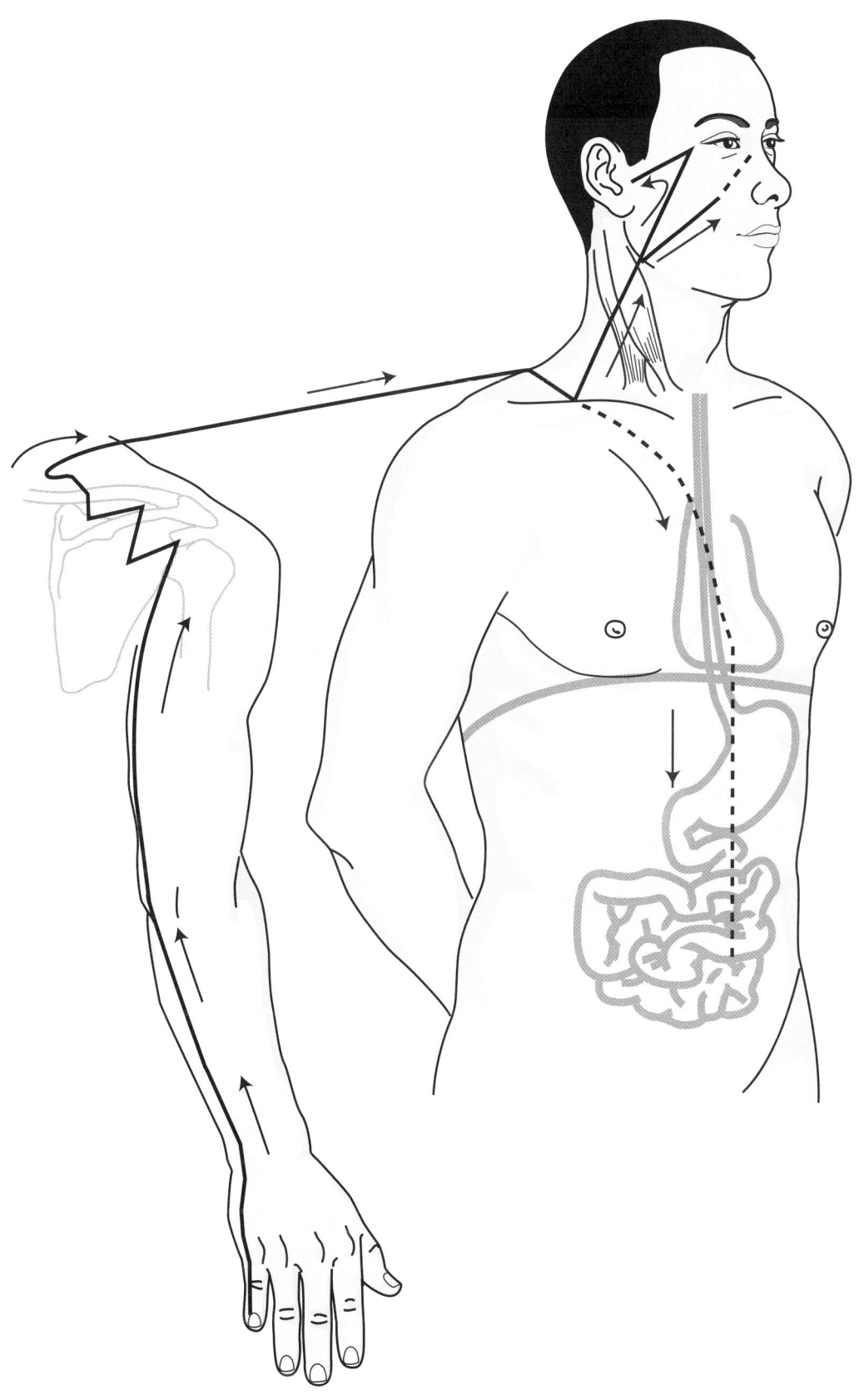

Figure 6.2 Small Intestine Channel — Stage 2

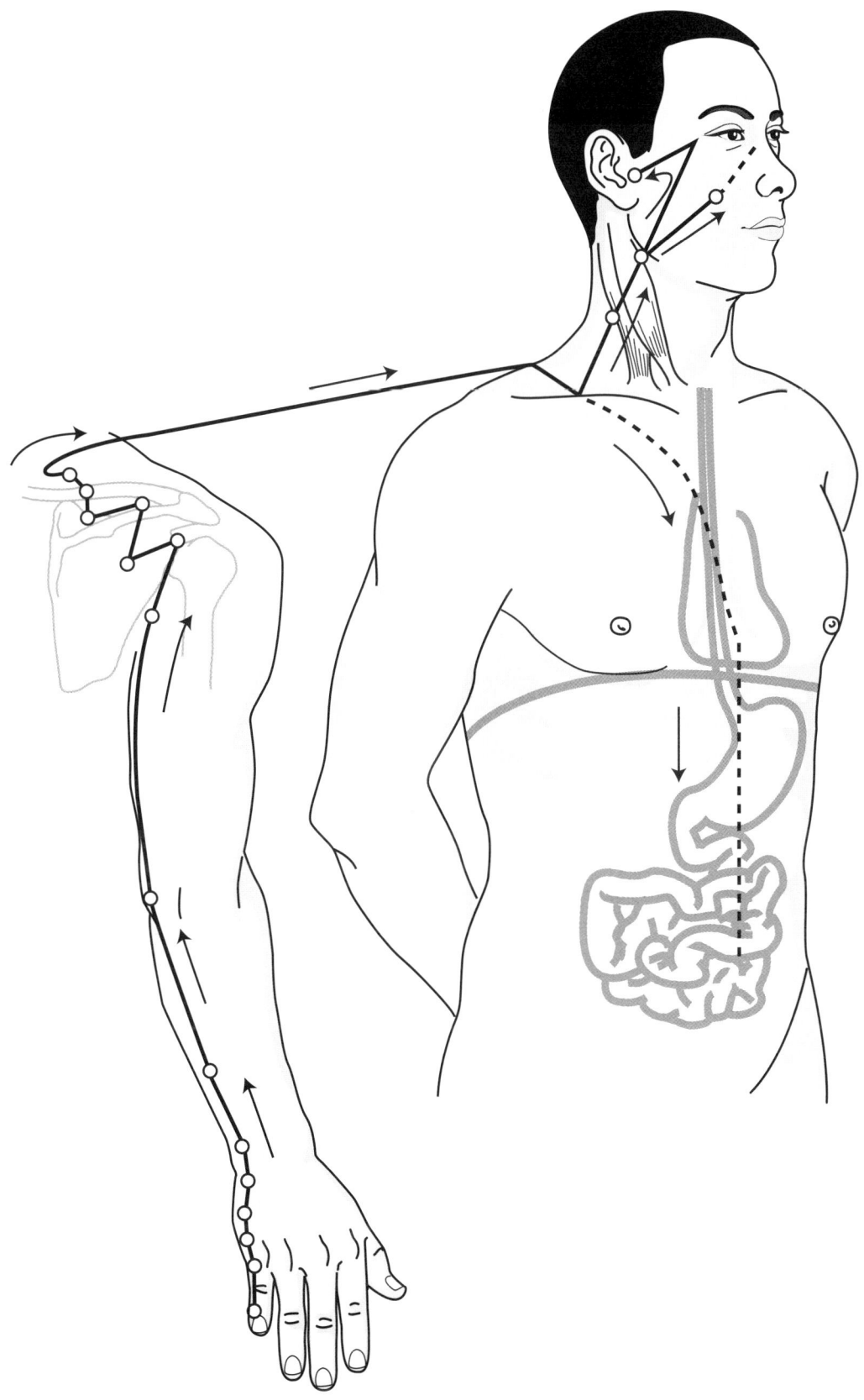

Figure 6.3 Small Intestine Channel — Stage 3

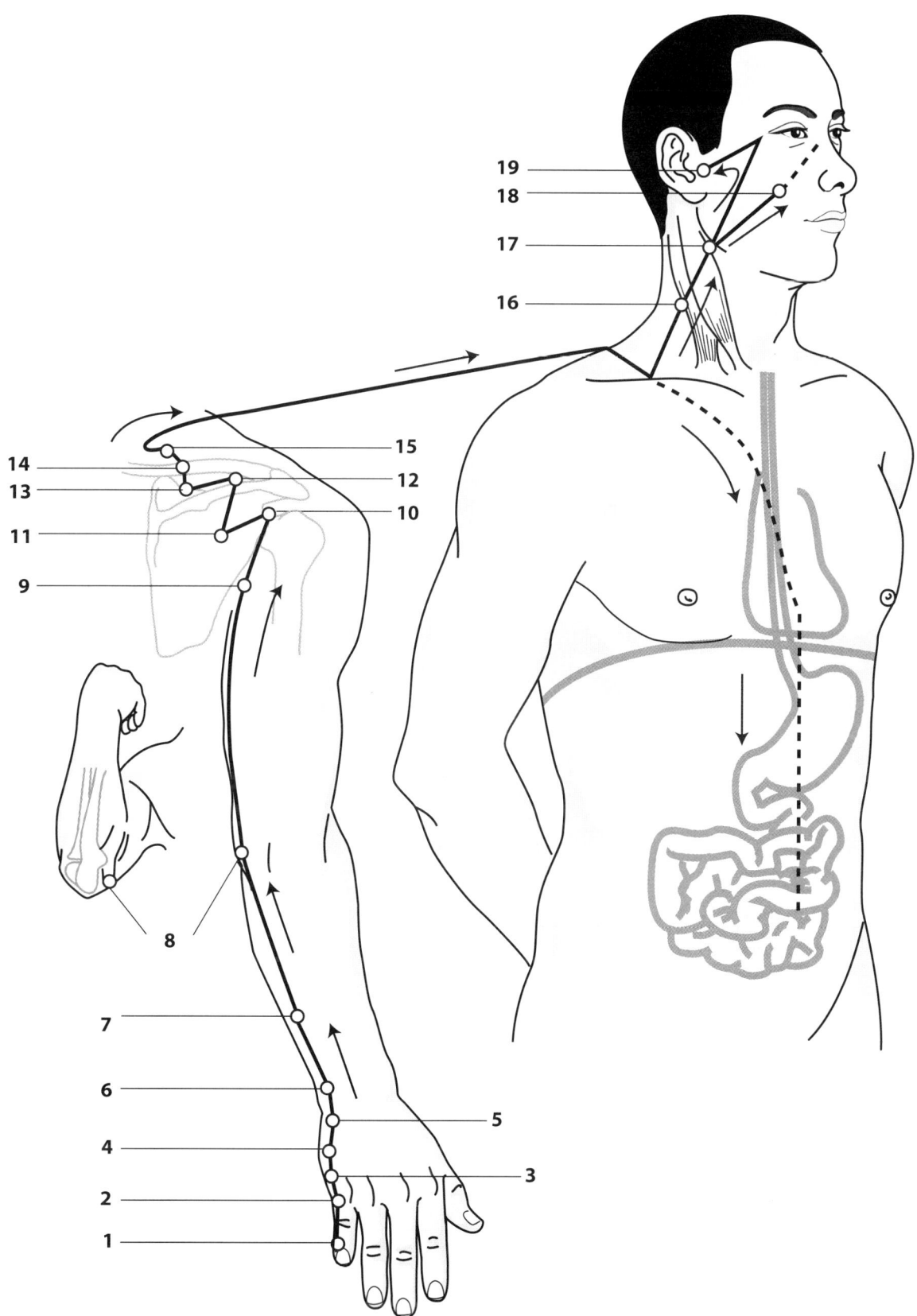

Figure 6.4 Small Intestine Channel — Stage 4

yuan — blue
luo — red
xi-cleft — green
five shu — yellow
lower he-sea — orange
back-shu — purple

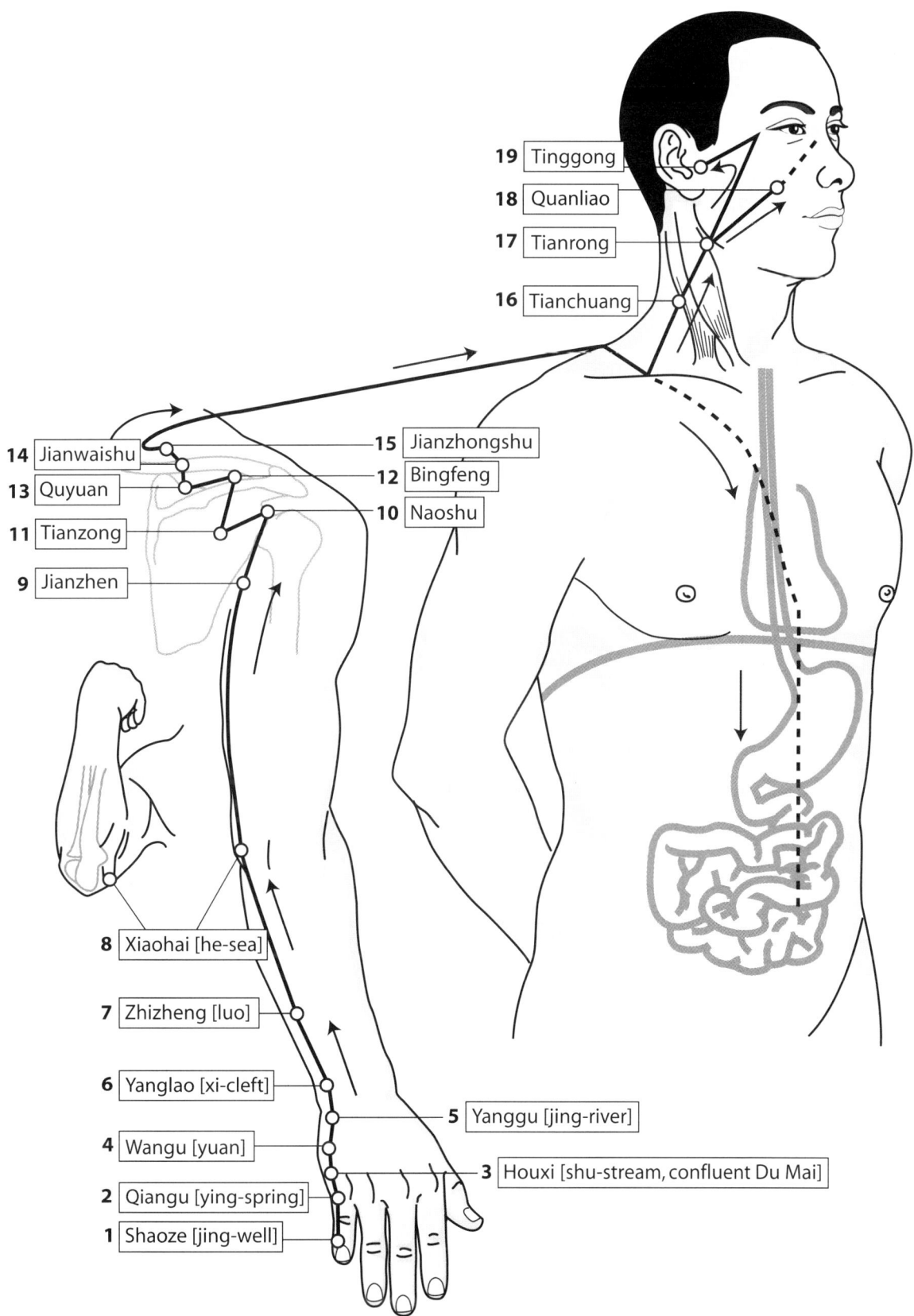

19 Tinggong

18 Quanliao

17 Tianrong

16 Tianchuang

14 Jianwaishu

13 Quyuan

11 Tianzong

9 Jianzhen

15 Jianzhongshu

12 Bingfeng

10 Naoshu

8 Xiaohai [he-sea]

7 Zhizheng [luo]

6 Yanglao [xi-cleft]

5 Yanggu [jing-river]

4 Wangu [yuan]

3 Houxi [shu-stream, confluent Du Mai]

2 Qiangu [ying-spring]

1 Shaoze [jing-well]

Figure 6.5 Small Intestine Channel — Stage 5

THE SMALL INTESTINE CHANNEL — CASE STUDY

Mr SB, 40 year old manager

Mr SB presents with an acute wry neck. On the previous day he was watching his son play rugby and standing with his back to a cold wind blowing across the field. This morning he woke with a painful 'locked neck' and now complains of stabbing pain and stiffness (8/10) on the right side of the neck radiating into the upper back and shoulder. The area is tender to touch and he has difficulty trying to turn his head. The pain is better for warmth, and worse for cold, wind or movement. He also complains of a runny nose with clear nasal discharge, and lack of perspiration.

QUESTIONS

Circle or write your answers as required.

1   Is this an external or internal disorder?

2   If external:

   (a) Is it due to heat or cold?

   (b) Are there symptoms of wind, dampness or dryness?

   (c) Is it acute, chronic or a mixed condition?

3   If internal:

   (a) Is it due to deficiency or excess?

      (i)   If deficient, is it: qi, blood, jin ye, yin or yang?

      (ii) If excess, is it: stagnant qi, stagnant blood, damp/phlegm, rebellious qi, rising liver yang, empty fire etc?

   (b) Is it due to cold or heat?

   (c) Which zang fu are affected?

   (d) Which channels are affected?

4 What might the pulse feel like?
   Describe: pulse rate, rhythm, depth, shape and strength.

5 What might the tongue look like?
   Describe:
   – tongue body (colour, shape, thickness)
   – tongue coating (moisture, colour, thickness, distribution, root).

6 What is the Chinese diagnosis?
   Where appropriate discuss the root (ben), the presenting symptoms (biao) and the five phase/ wu xing dynamics (the relationship between and among the zang fu organs under syndromes of imbalance or disease).

7 What is your treatment principle?

8 What points would you use and why? Include adjunctive therapy such as moxa or cupping if appropriate.
   (A minimum of five points, use only points on the Lung, Large Intestine, Stomach, Spleen, Heart and Small Intestine Channels.)

Chapter Seven

THE BLADDER CHANNEL OF FOOT TAIYANG AND BACK-SHU POINTS

足太阳膀胱经和背俞穴

The Bladder Channel of Foot Taiyang is *biao li* partnered with the Kidney Channel and paired with the Small Intestine Channel according to six channel theory.

The use of the Bladder Channel is based on knowing the functions and indications of the Bladder Channel points and the pathophysiology of the bladder as a *fu*.

The Bladder Channel connects with the following zang fu:

Kidney   Bladder

The main pathway:

- begins at the inner canthus of the eye at Jingming BL1

- ascends over the forehead joining Du Mai at the vertex at Baihui Du20

- from the vertex, the main branch enters the brain, intersects with Du Mai at Naohu Du17, then emerges and splits into two branches at the nape of the neck

- at the nape of the neck, the medial branch runs downward 1.5 cun parallel to the vertebral column until it reaches the lumbar region where a branch enters the body (see other branches)

- the medial branch continues down along the sacrum, crosses the buttock and descends to the popliteal fossa of the knee

- the lateral branch runs down from the neck 3 cun parallel to the spine until it reaches the gluteal region where it crosses the buttock and intersects with the Gall Bladder Channel at Huantiao GB30

- descends along the postero-lateral aspect of the thigh to meet with the medial branch in the popliteal fossa

- the two branches merge and the channel descends through the gastrocnemius muscle to the lateral malleolus

- runs along the fifth metatarsal until it reaches the lateral side of the tip of the little toe at Zhiyin BL67, where it meets with the Kidney Channel.

The other branches:

- from the vertex at Baihui Du20, a branch descends to the temple to intersect with and follow the Gall Bladder points around the ear

- in the lumbar region the channel enters the body cavity via the paravertebral muscles to connect with the kidney and the bladder.

The Bladder Channel connects with other primary channels at various points on the body, specifically Du Mai and Gall Bladder Channels, and also Large Intestine and Small Intestine Channels (not always shown in diagrams).

THE BLADDER CHANNEL POINTS

WHO number	Pinyin	Name	Specific functions
BL1	**Jingming**	Bright Eyes	
BL2	**Zanzhu**	Bamboo Gathering	
BL3	Meichong	Eyebrow Ascension	
BL4	Quchai	Deviating Turn	
BL5	Wuchu	Fifth Place	
BL6	Chengguang	Light Guard	
BL7	**Tongtian**	Celestial Collection	
BL8	Luoque	Declining Connection	
BL9	Yuzhen	Jade Pillow	
BL10	**Tianzhu**	Celestial Pillar	
BL11	**Dazhu**	Great Shuttle	Influential Point of Bone
BL12	**Fengmen**	Wind Gate	
BL13	**Feishu**	Lung Shu	Back-Shu (LU)
BL14	**Jueyinshu**	Jueyinshu	Back-Shu (PC)
BL15	**Xinshu**	Heart Shu	Back-Shu (HT)
BL16	Dushu	Governing Shu	
BL17	**Geshu**	Diaphragm Shu	Influential Point of Blood
BL18	**Ganshu**	Liver Shu	Back-Shu (LR)
BL19	**Danshu**	Gall Bladder Shu	Back-Shu (GB)
BL20	**Pishu**	Spleen Shu	Back-Shu (SP)
BL21	**Weishu**	Stomach Shu	Back-Shu (ST)
BL22	**Sanjiaoshu**	Sanjiao Shu	Back-Shu (SJ)
BL23	**Shenshu**	Kidney Shu	Back-Shu (KI)
BL24	**Qihaishu**	Sea-of-Qi Shu	
BL25	**Dachangshu**	Large Intestine Shu	Back-Shu (LI)
BL26	**Guanyuanshu**	Origin Pass Shu	
BL27	**Xiaochangshu**	Small Intestine Shu	Back-Shu (SI)
BL28	**Pangguangshu**	Bladder Shu	Back-Shu (BL)
BL29	Zhonglushu	Central Backbone Shu	
BL30	**Baihuanshu**	White Ring Shu	
BL31	**Shangliao**	Upper Bone-Hole	
BL32	**Ciliao**	Second Bone-Hole	
BL33	**Zhongliao**	Central Bone-Hole	
BL34	**Xialiao**	Lower Bone-Hole	
BL35	**Huiyang**	Meeting of Yang	
BL36	**Chengfu**	Support	

WHO number	Pinyin	Name	Specific functions
BL37	**Yinmen**	Gate of Abundance	
BL38	**Fuxi**	Superficial Cleft	
BL39	**Weiyang**	Bend Yang	Lower He-Sea (SJ)
BL40	**Weizhong**	Bend Middle	He-Sea*5
BL41	Fufen	Attached Branch	
BL42	**Pohu**	Po Door	
BL43	**Gaohuangshu**	Gao Huang Shu	
BL44	**Shentang**	Spirit Hall	
BL45	Yixi	Yixi	
BL46	Geguan	Diaphragm Pass	
BL47	**Hunmen**	Hun Gate	
BL48	Yanggang	Yang Head Rope	
BL49	**Yishe**	Reflection Abode	
BL50	Weicang	Stomach Granary	
BL51	**Huangmen**	Huang Gate	
BL52	**Zhishi**	Will Chamber	
BL53	**Baohuang**	Bladder Huang	
BL54	**Zhibian**	Sequential Limit	
BL55	Heyang	Yang Union	
BL56	Chengjin	Sinew Support	
BL57	**Chengshan**	Mountain Support	
BL58	**Feiyang**	Taking Flight	Luo-Connecting
BL59	**Fuyang**	Instep Yang	Xi-Cleft Yangqiao Mai
BL60	**Kunlun**	Kunlun Mountains	Jing-River*4
BL61	**Pucan**	Subservient Visitor	
BL62	**Shenmai**	Extending Vessel	Confluent Yangqiao Mai
BL63	**Jinmen**	Metal Gate	Xi-Cleft
BL64	**Jinggu**	Capital Bone	Yuan-Source
BL65	**Shugu**	Bundle Bone	Shu-Stream*3
BL66	**Zutonggu**	Foot Valley Passage	Ying-Spring*2
BL67	**Zhiyin**	Reaching Yin	Jing-Well*1

* The 5 Shu points of the Yang Channels:
      1 = metal
      2 = water
      3 = wood
      4 = fire
      5 = earth

Note: The 52 points highlighted in bold are provided on the composite diagram for this channel (the fifth diagram).

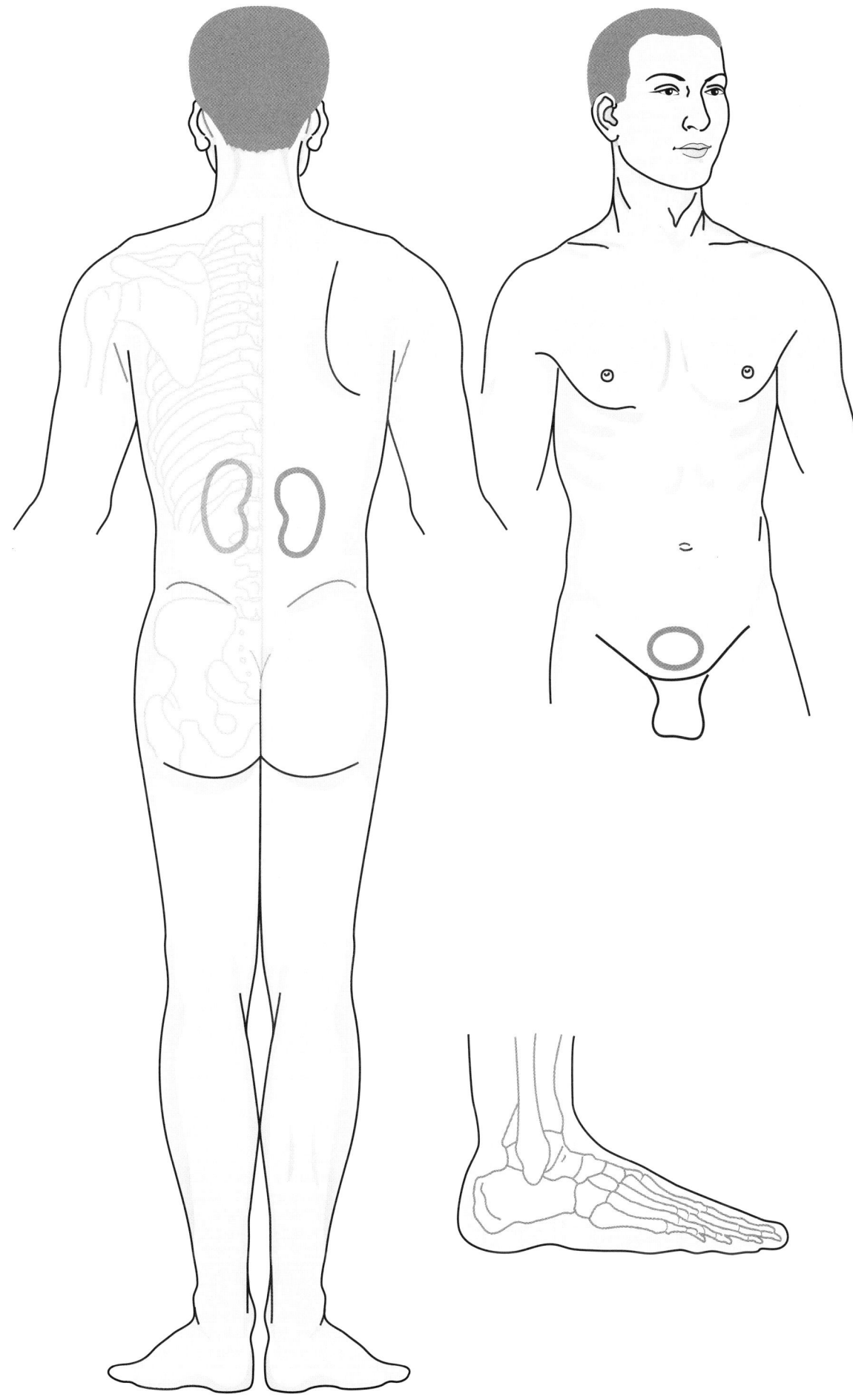

Figure 7.1 Bladder Channel — Stage 1

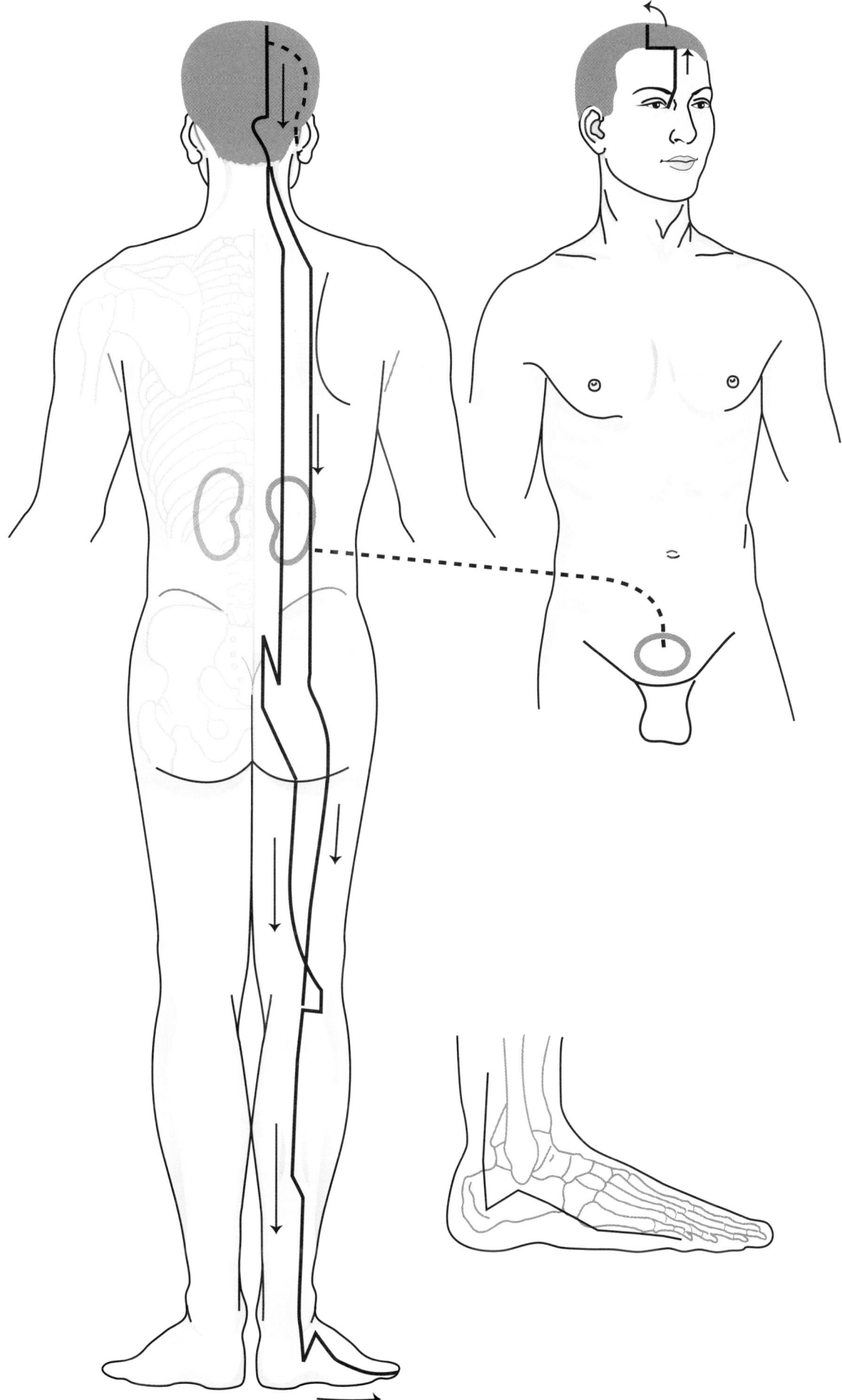

Figure 7.2 Bladder Channel — Stage 2

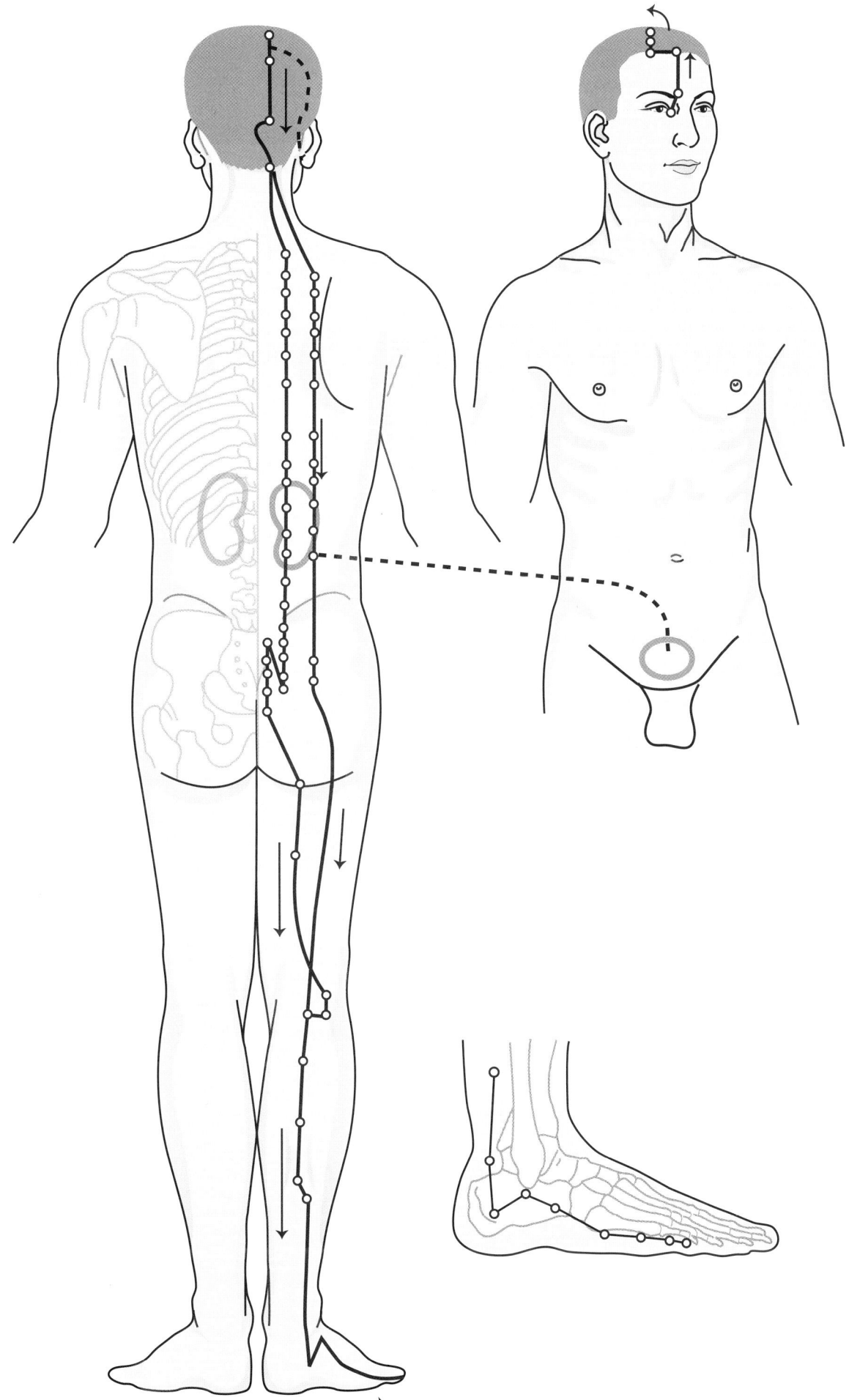

Figure 7.3 Bladder Channel — Stage 3

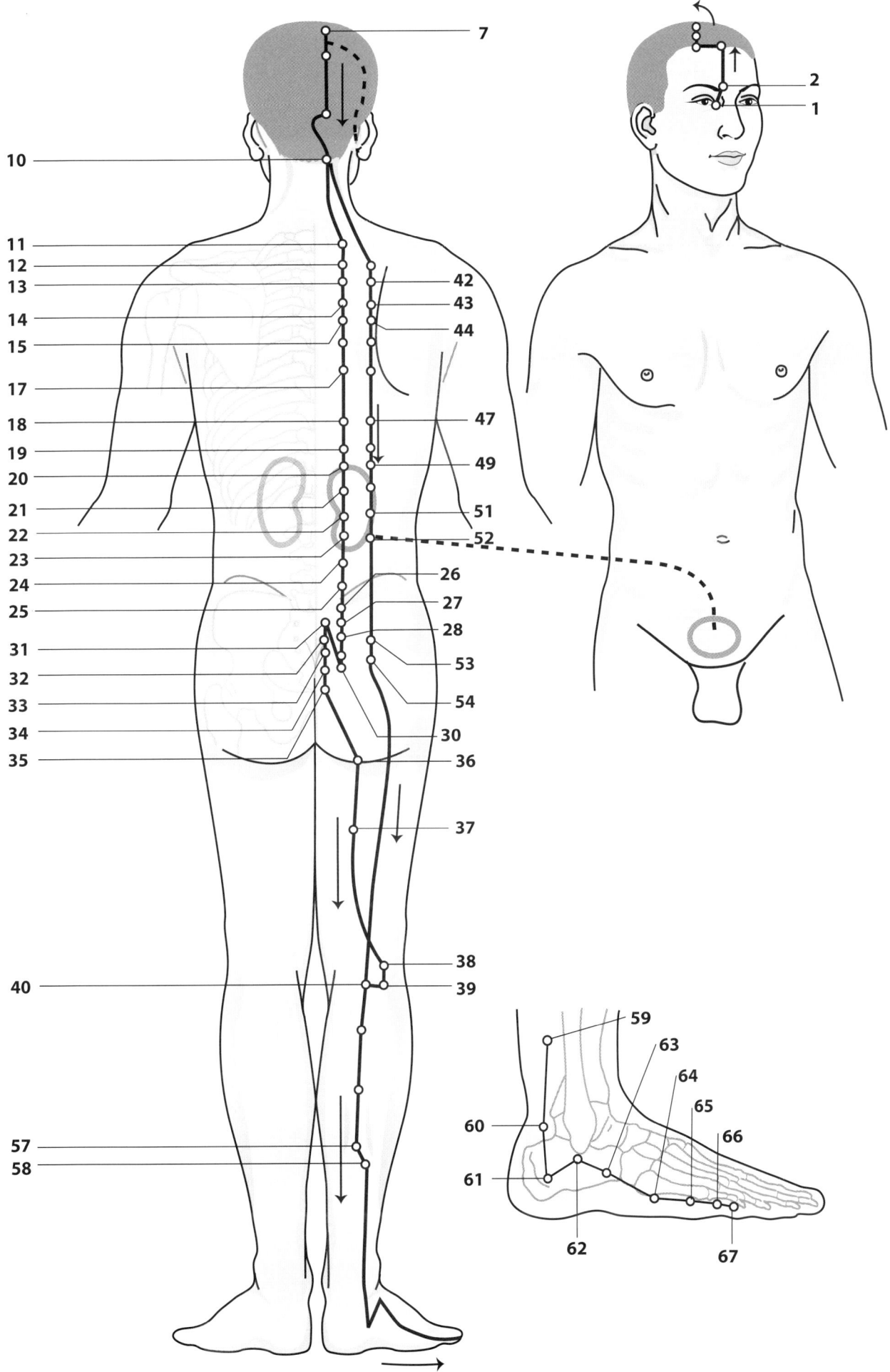

Figure 7.4 Bladder Channel — Stage 4

yuan — blue	
luo — red	
xi-cleft — green	
five shu — yellow	
lower he-sea — orange	
back-shu — purple	

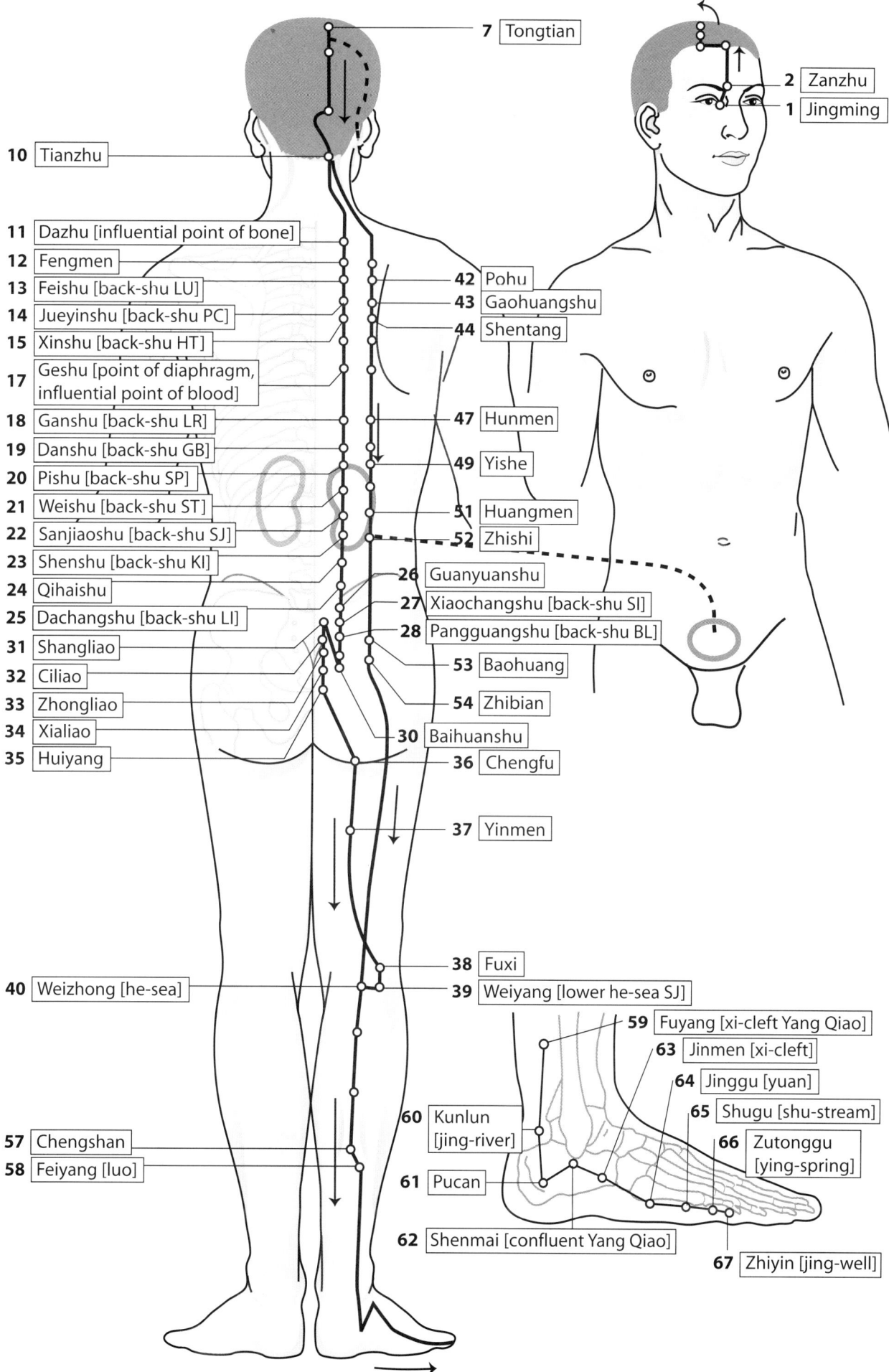

7 Tongtian
2 Zanzhu
1 Jingming
10 Tianzhu
11 Dazhu [influential point of bone]
12 Fengmen
13 Feishu [back-shu LU]
14 Jueyinshu [back-shu PC]
15 Xinshu [back-shu HT]
17 Geshu [point of diaphragm, influential point of blood]
18 Ganshu [back-shu LR]
19 Danshu [back-shu GB]
20 Pishu [back-shu SP]
21 Weishu [back-shu ST]
22 Sanjiaoshu [back-shu SJ]
23 Shenshu [back-shu KI]
24 Qihaishu
25 Dachangshu [back-shu LI]
31 Shangliao
32 Ciliao
33 Zhongliao
34 Xialiao
35 Huiyang
42 Pohu
43 Gaohuangshu
44 Shentang
47 Hunmen
49 Yishe
51 Huangmen
52 Zhishi
26 Guanyuanshu
27 Xiaochangshu [back-shu SI]
28 Pangguangshu [back-shu BL]
53 Baohuang
54 Zhibian
30 Baihuanshu
36 Chengfu
37 Yinmen
38 Fuxi
40 Weizhong [he-sea]
39 Weiyang [lower he-sea SJ]
59 Fuyang [xi-cleft Yang Qiao]
63 Jinmen [xi-cleft]
64 Jinggu [yuan]
60 Kunlun [jing-river]
65 Shugu [shu-stream]
66 Zutonggu [ying-spring]
57 Chengshan
58 Feiyang [luo]
61 Pucan
62 Shenmai [confluent Yang Qiao]
67 Zhiyin [jing-well]

Figure 7.5 Bladder Channel — Stage 5

Back-Shu Points

These points lie along the Bladder Channel (*yang*) and are situated close to their respective *zang fu* organs. They are specific points where the *qi* of the *zang fu* involved is infused. They are invaluable for disorders of the internal organs.

On the front of the body, at roughly the same anatomical location, are a series of points known as the 'front-*mu* points'. These points are *yin*, and diseases of the fu organs (*yang*) manifest in them. Use them to treat problems of the six *fu*. These have also been included for your reference.

BACK SHU CHANNEL POINTS AND FRONT MU CHANNEL POINTS			
Organ	Shu	Mu	Scope of Treatment
LU	BL13 Feishu	LU1 Zhongfu	Respiratory system disorders such as cough, dyspnoea, thoracic fullness and distension
PC	BL14 Jueyinshu	CV17 Shanzong	Heart illnesses such as cardiac pain and palpitations
HT	BL15 Xinshu	CV14 Juque	Heart and stomach disorders such as palpitations, stomach pain and neurasthenia
LR	BL18 Ganshu	LR14 Qimen	Liver and stomach disorders such as liver region pain, vomiting and regurgitation of acid fluid
GB	BL19 Danshu	GB24 Riyue	Liver and gall bladder disorders such as pain in the area of Riyue GB24 and jaundice
SP	BL20 Pishu	LR13 Zhangmen	Liver and spleen disorders such as enlargement or pain in either organ, abdominal pain or distension, and poor digestion
ST	BL21 Weishu	CV12* Zhongwan	Stomach region disorders such as stomach pain or distension and lack of appetite
SJ	BL22 Sanjiaoshu	CV5 Shimen	Water metabolism dysfunction such as oedema, ascites and diarrhoea
KI	BL23 Shenshu	GB25 Jingmen	Kidney and urogenital disorders, low back pain or soreness, seminal loss, and premature ejaculation
LI	BL25 Dachangshu	ST25 Tianshu	Large intestine disorders such as constipation, diarrhoea and abdominal pain
SI	BL27 Xiaochangshu	CV4 Guanyuan	Small intestine, bladder and urogenital disorders such as gripping intestinal pain, shan qi, enuresis, urinary obstruction and seminal loss
BL	BL28 Pangguangshu	CV3 Zhongji	Bladder and urogenital disorders such as enuresis, urinary block, seminal loss, and menstrual disorders

*Zhizheng SI7 is listed in some older texts as the front-*mu* point of the stomach.

The back-*shu* and front-*mu* points are points on the torso that directly affect a related *zang* or *fu* organ, despite the channel they are on. Traditionally the back-*shu* points, being *yang*, were used for draining excess, and the front-*mu*, being *yin*, were used to tonify deficiency.

Another theory proposed the back-*shu* points were best to treat the yin *zang* organs, while the front-*shu* points best treated the *yang fu* organs. Today the back-*shu* are used for either tonification or dispersion although the front-*mu* are generally used for tonification. Corresponding back-*shu* and front-*mu* are often combined.

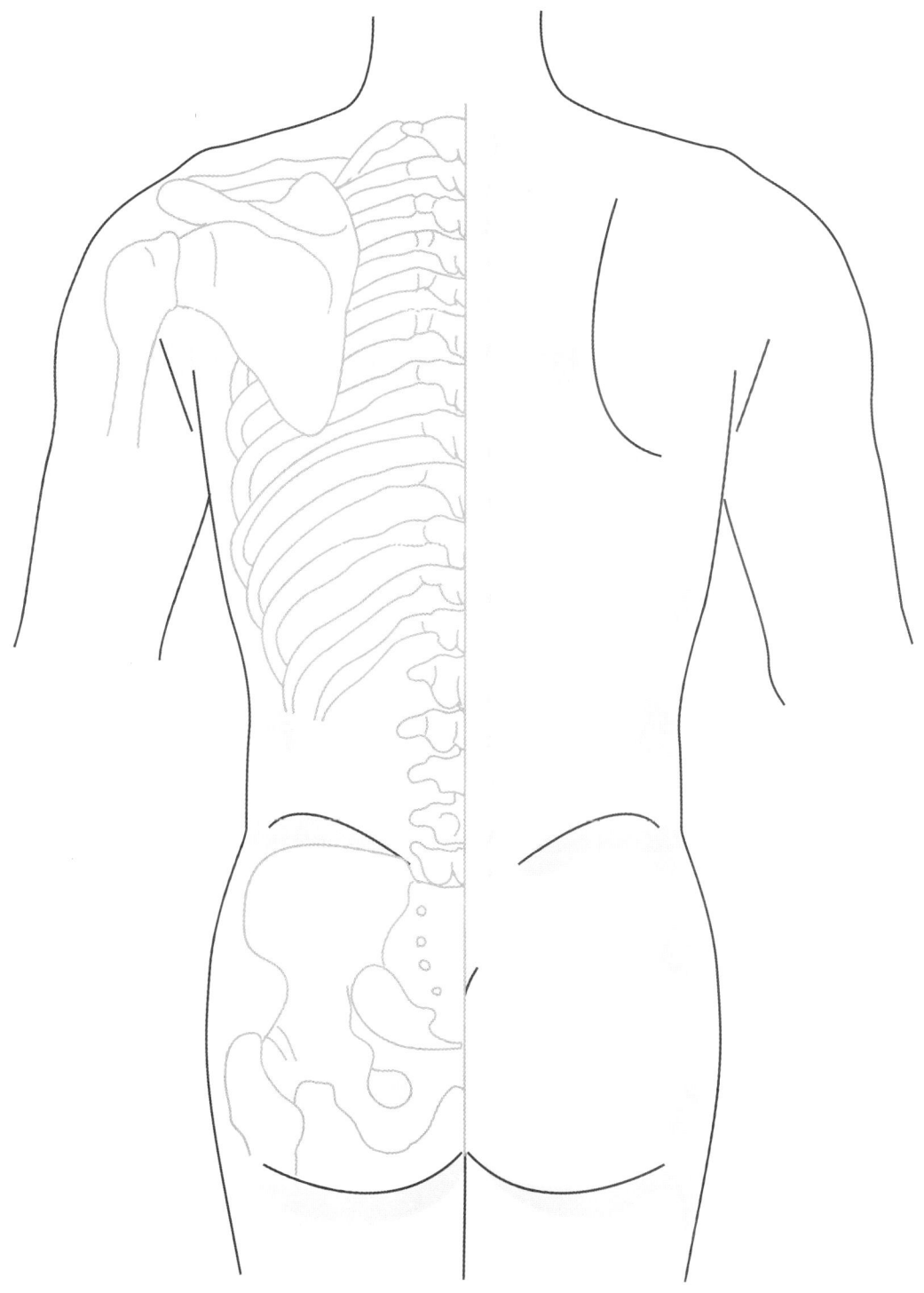

Figure 7.6 Back-Shu Points — Stage 1

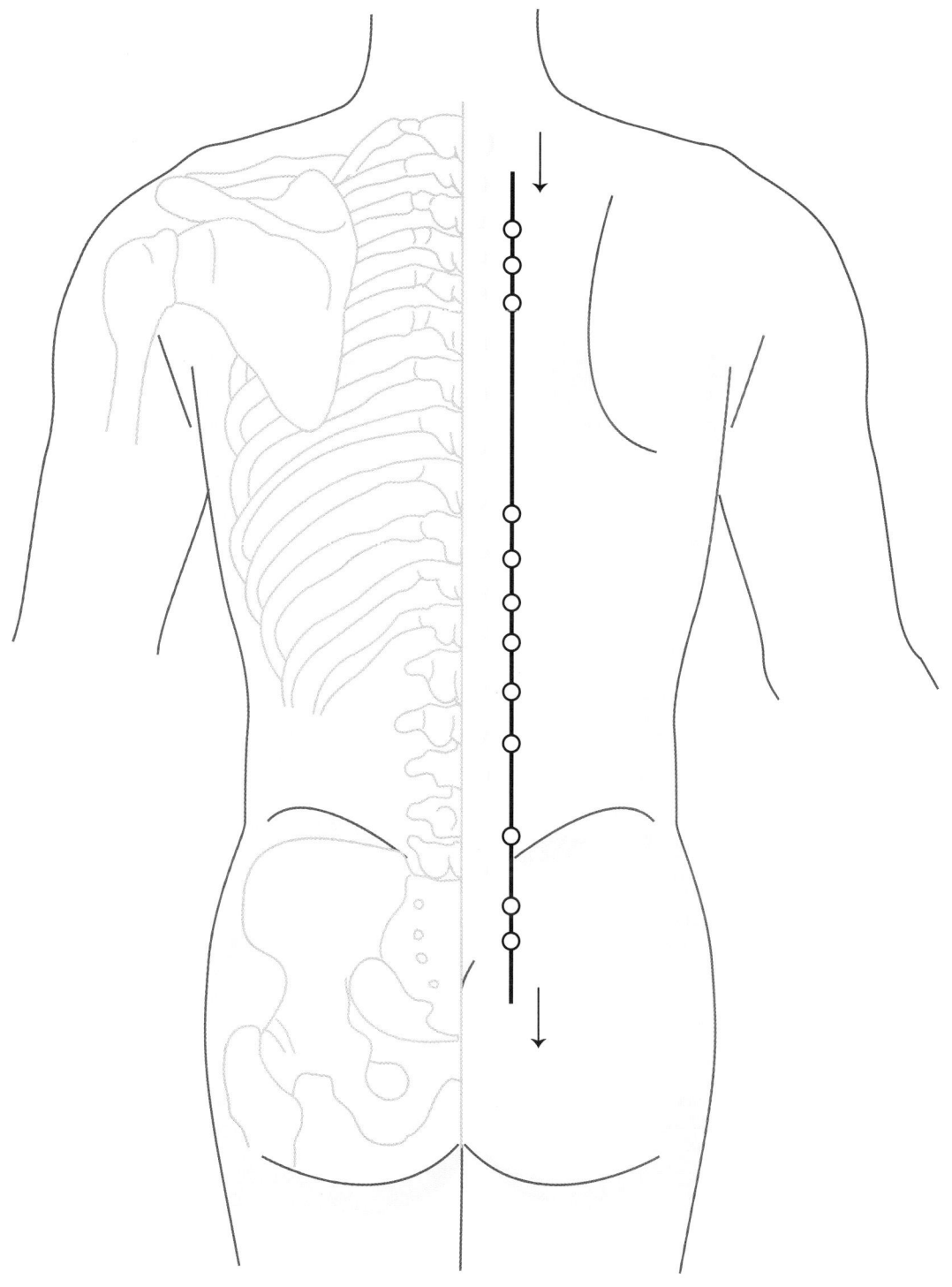

Figure 7.7 Back-Shu Points — Stage 2

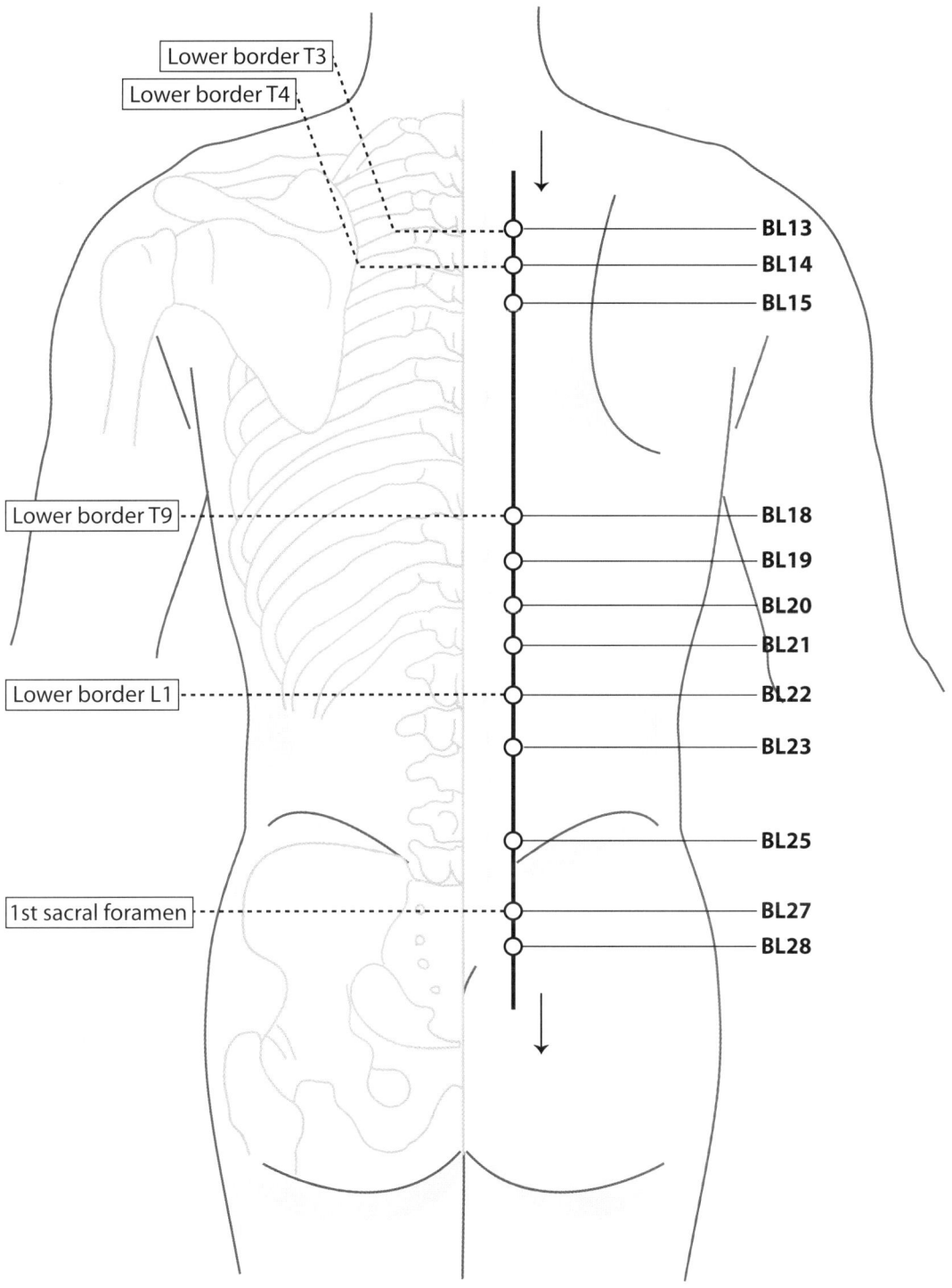

Figure 7.8 Back-Shu Points — Stage 3

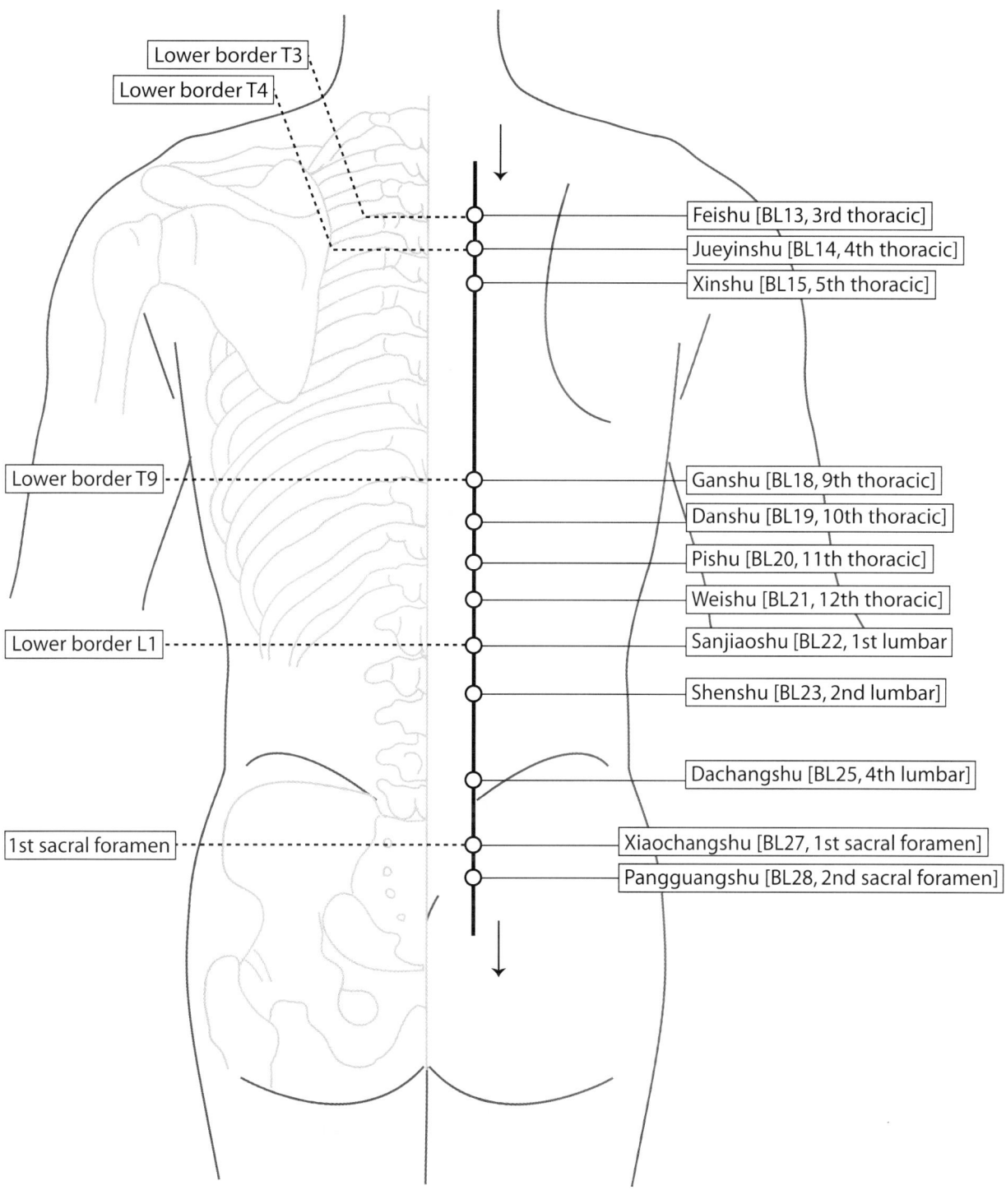

Lower border T3

Lower border T4

Feishu [BL13, 3rd thoracic]

Jueyinshu [BL14, 4th thoracic]

Xinshu [BL15, 5th thoracic]

Lower border T9

Ganshu [BL18, 9th thoracic]

Danshu [BL19, 10th thoracic]

Pishu [BL20, 11th thoracic]

Weishu [BL21, 12th thoracic]

Lower border L1

Sanjiaoshu [BL22, 1st lumbar]

Shenshu [BL23, 2nd lumbar]

Dachangshu [BL25, 4th lumbar]

1st sacral foramen

Xiaochangshu [BL27, 1st sacral foramen]

Pangguangshu [BL28, 2nd sacral foramen]

Figure 7.9 Back-Shu Points — Stage 4

THE BLADDER CHANNEL — CASE STUDY

Miss SO, 22 year old office worker

Miss SO has recently returned from a holiday in Malaysia where she has been exposed to damp sticky weather. She presents with painful, burning and frequent urination, a sense of urgency, dark yellow urine and occasionally some blood in her early morning urine. She also complains of feeling hot and being thirsty.

QUESTIONS

Circle or write your answers as required.

1 Is this an external or internal disorder?

2 If external:
   (a) Is it due to heat or cold?

   (b) Are there symptoms of wind, dampness or dryness?

   (c) Is it acute, chronic or a mixed condition?

3 If internal:
   (a) Is it due to deficiency or excess?

       (i)   If deficient, is it: qi, blood, jin ye, yin or yang?

       (ii) If excess, is it: stagnant qi, stagnant blood, damp/phlegm, rebellious qi, rising liver yang, empty fire etc?

   (b) Is it due to cold or heat?

   (c) Which zang fu are affected?

   (d) Which channels are affected?

4 **What might the pulse feel like?**
   Describe: pulse rate, rhythm, depth, shape and strength.

5 **What might the tongue look like?**
   Describe:
   – tongue body (colour, shape, thickness)
   – tongue coating (moisture, colour, thickness, distribution, root).

6 **What is the Chinese diagnosis?**
   Where appropriate discuss the root (ben), the presenting symptoms (biao) and the five phase/ wu xing dynamics (the relationship between and among the zang fu organs under syndromes of imbalance or disease).

7 **What is your treatment principle?**

8 **What points would you use and why? Include adjunctive therapy such as moxa or cupping, if appropriate.**
   (A minimum of five points, use only points on the Lung, Large Intestine, Stomach, Spleen, Heart, Small Intestine and Bladder Channels.)

Chapter Eight

THE KIDNEY CHANNEL OF FOOT SHAOYIN

足少阴肾经

The Kidney Channel of Foot Shaoyin is *biao li* partnered with the Bladder Channel and paired with the Heart Channel according to six channel theory.

The use of the Kidney Channel is based on knowing the functions and indications of the Kidney Channel points and the pathophysiology of the kidney as a *zang*.

The Kidney Channel connects with the following zang fu:

Kidney   Bladder   Liver   Lung   Heart

The main pathway:

- begins underneath the little toe and runs obliquely across the sole of the foot through Yongquan KI1 to emerge anterior and inferior to the navicular tuberosity

- travels posterior to the medial malleolus, loops down through the heel, then ascends to below the medial malleolus

- runs up the medial aspect of the leg to the medial side of the popliteal fossa

- continues up along the postero-medial aspect of the thigh to the tip of the coccyx where it intersects with Du Mai at Changqiang Du1 (see other branches)

- re-emerges at the superior border of the symphysis pubis, then intersects with Ren Mai in the lower abdomen

- ascends 0.5 cun lateral to the midline until it reaches Youmen KI21, 6 cun above the umbilicus

- ascends 2 cun lateral to the midline from the fifth to the first intercostal space

- ends in the depression on the lower border of the clavicle at Shufu KI27.

The other branches:

- a branch begins at the coccyx and threads its way through the spine to enter the kidney and connect with the bladder

- a second branch emerges from the kidney, ascends through the liver and diaphragm, enters the lung, runs upward along the throat and ends at the root of the tongue

- another branch springs from the lung, joins with the heart and disperses in the chest to link with the Pericardium Channel of Hand Jueyin at Shanzhong Ren17.

The Kidney Channel connects with other primary channels at various points on the body, specifically the Spleen, Du Mai and Ren Mai Channels.

THE KIDNEY CHANNEL POINTS			
WHO number	**Pinyin**	**Name**	**Specific functions**
KI1	**Yongquan**	Gushing Spring	Jing-Well*1
KI2	**Rangu**	Blazing Valley	Ying-Spring*2
KI3	**Taixi**	Great Ravine	Yuan-Source, Shu-Stream*3
KI4	**Dazhong**	Large Goblet	Luo-Connecting
KI5	**Shuiquan**	Water Spring	Xi-Cleft
KI6	**Zhaohai**	Shining Sea	Confluent Yin Qiao Mai
KI7	**Fuliu**	Recover Flow	Jing-River*4
KI8	**Jiaoxin**	Intersection Reach	Xi-Cleft Yin Qiao Mai
KI9	**Zhubin**	Guest House	Xi-Cleft Yin Wei Mai
KI10	**Yingu**	Yin Valley	He-Sea*5
KI11	**Henggu**	Pubic Bone	
KI12	**Dahe**	Great Manifestation	
KI13	**Qixue**	Qi Hole	
KI14	**Siman**	Fourfold Fullness	
KI15	Zhongzhu	Central Flow	
KI16	Huangshu	Huang Shu	
KI17	Shangqu	Shang Bend	
KI18	Shiguan	Stone Pass	
KI19	**Yindu**	Yin Metropolis	
KI20	Futonggu	Abdomen Open Valley	
KI21	**Youmen**	Dark Gate	
KI22	Bulang	Corridor Walk	
KI23	Shenfeng	Spirit Seal	
KI24	Lingxu	Spirit Ruins	
KI25	Shencang	Spirit Storehouse	
KI26	Yuzhong	Lively Centre	
KI27	**Shufu**	Shu Mansion	

* The 5 Shu points of the Yin Channels:

     1 = wood
     2 = fire
     3 = earth
     4 = metal
     5 = water

Note: The 17 points highlighted in bold are provided on the composite diagram for this channel (the fifth diagram).

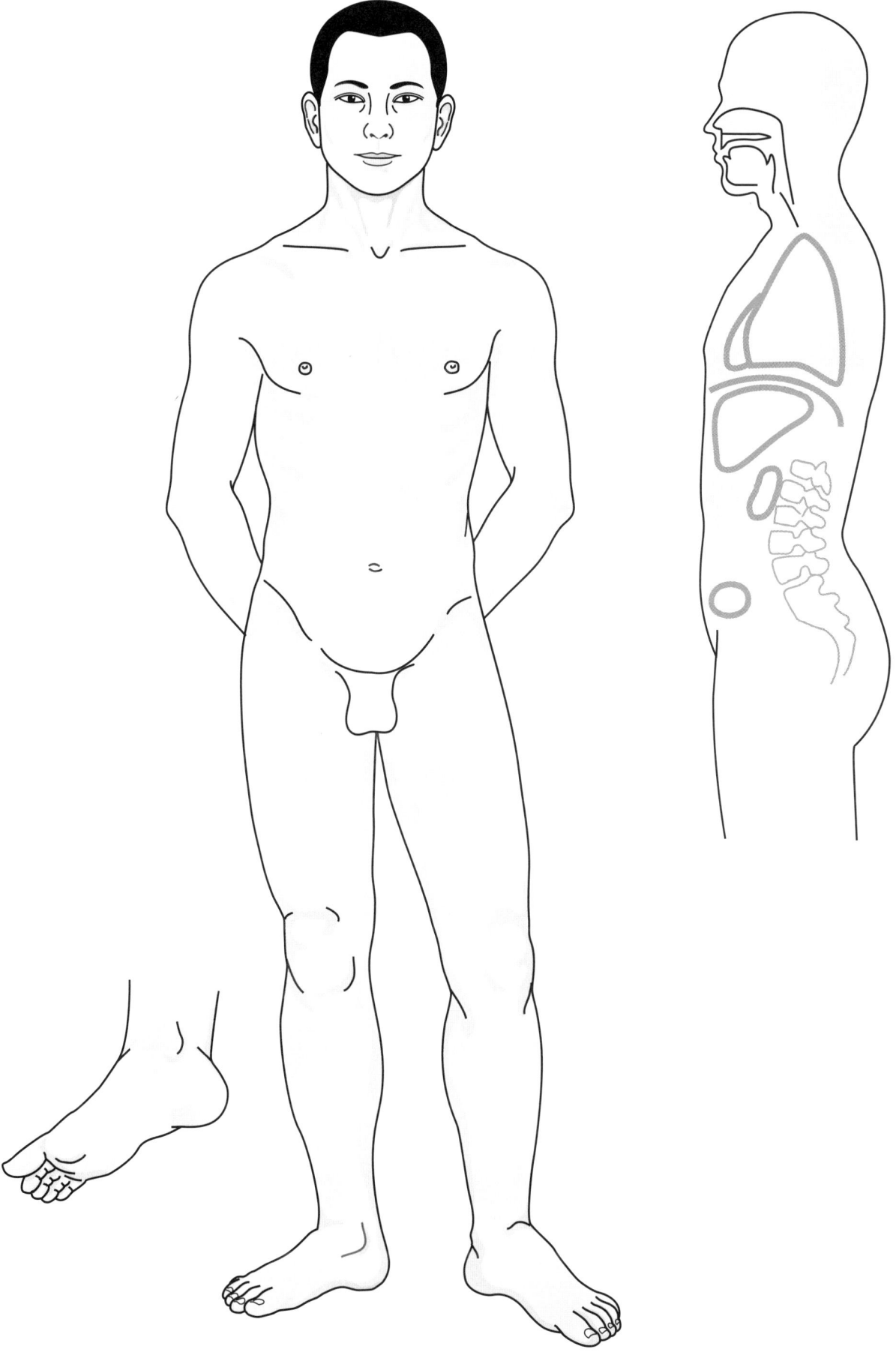

Figure 8.1 The Kidney Channel — Stage 1

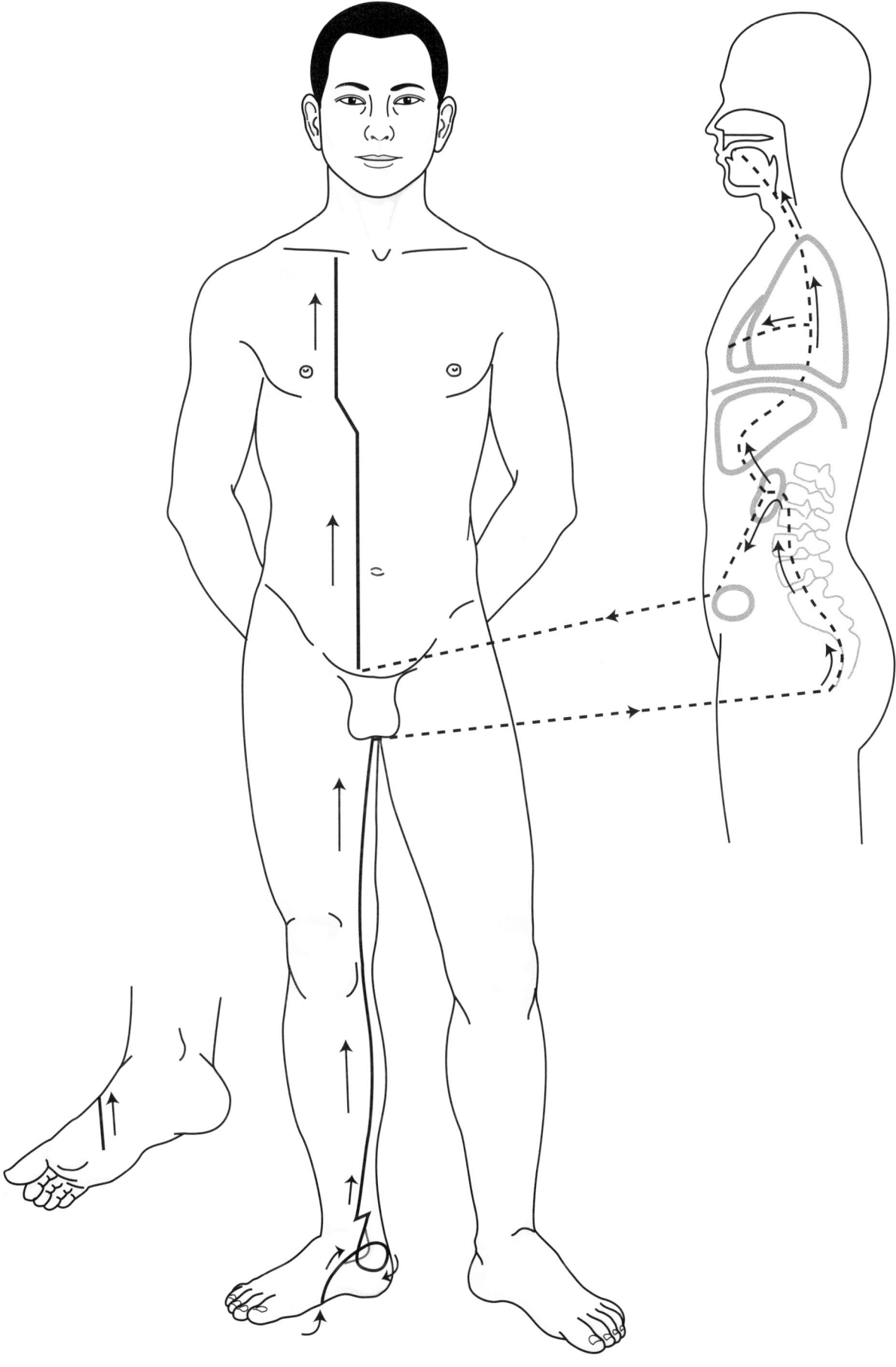

Figure 8.2 The Kidney Channel — Stage 2

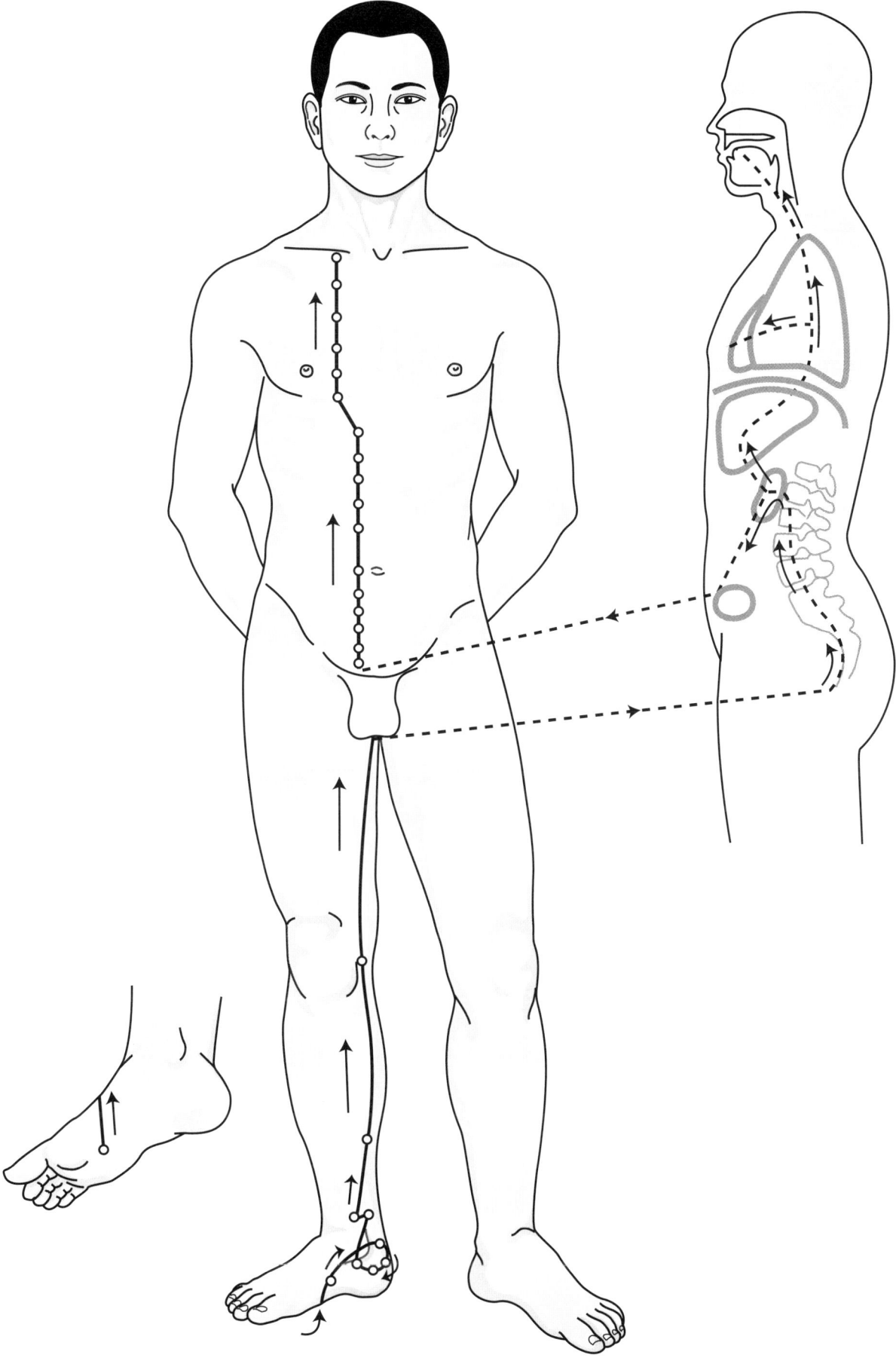

Figure 8.3 The Kidney Channel — Stage 3

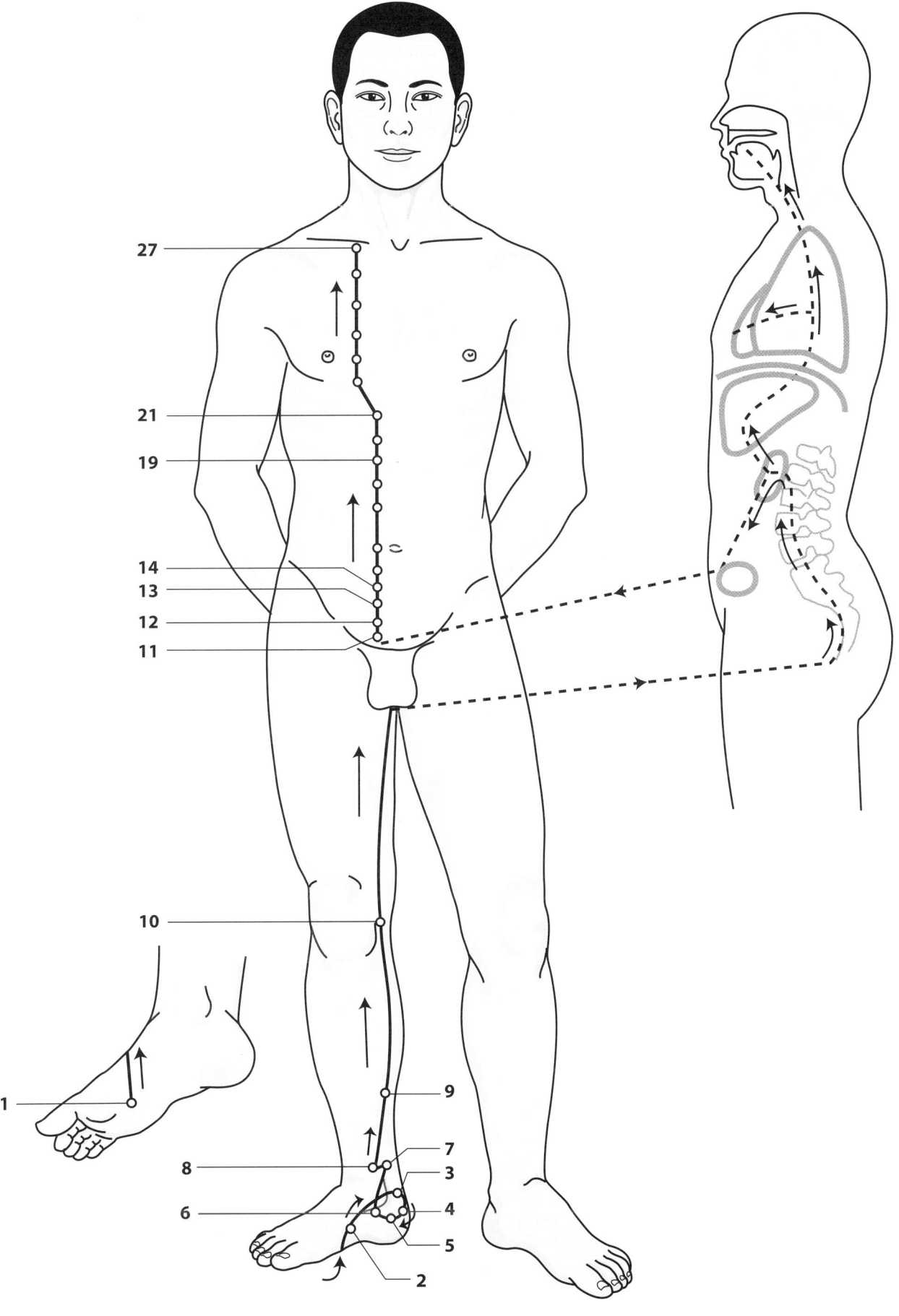

Figure 8.4 The Kidney Channel — Stage 4

yuan — blue	
luo — red	
xi-cleft — green	
five shu — yellow	
lower he-sea — orange	
back-shu — purple	

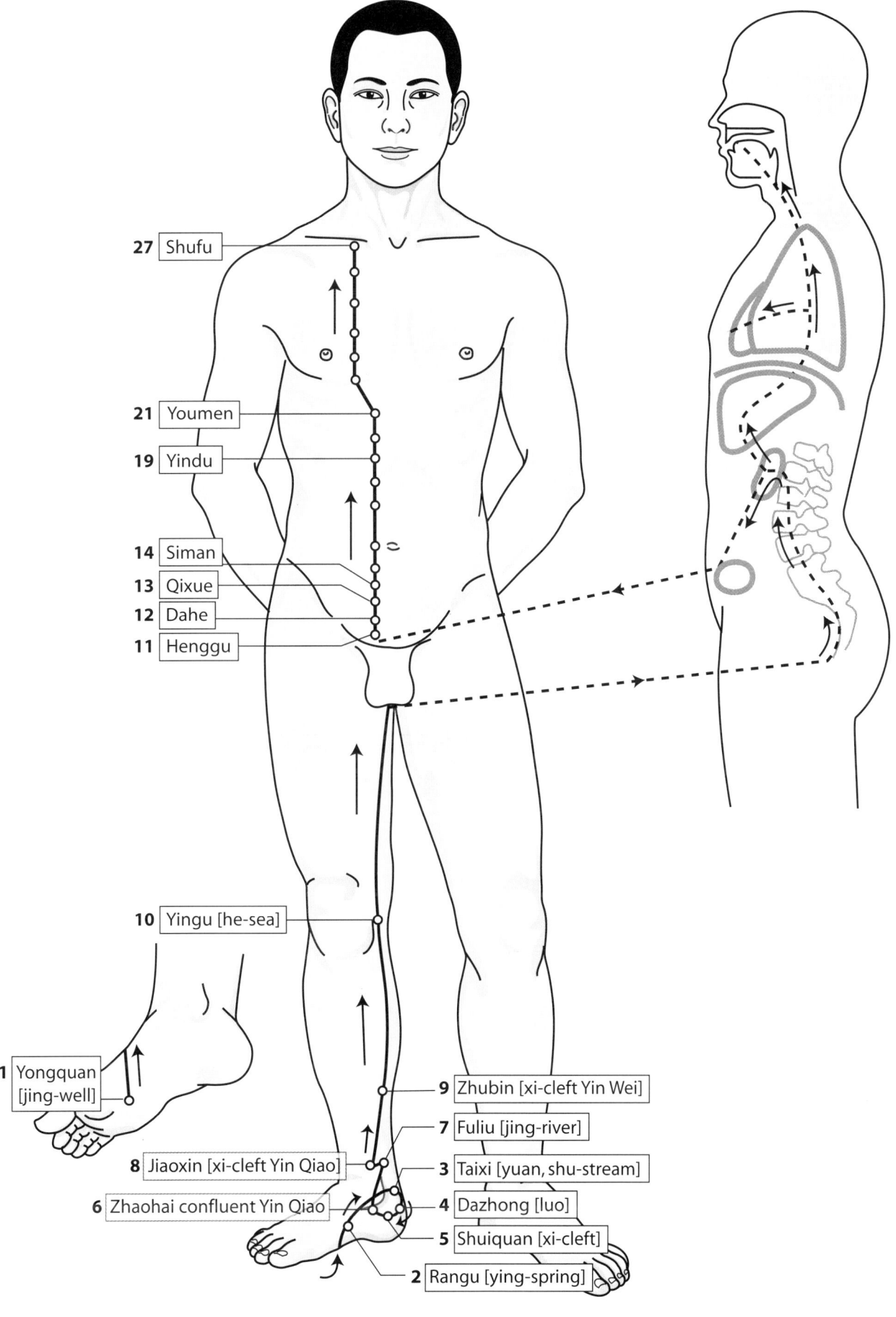

27 Shufu

21 Youmen

19 Yindu

14 Siman

13 Qixue

12 Dahe

11 Henggu

10 Yingu [he-sea]

1 Yongquan [jing-well]

8 Jiaoxin [xi-cleft Yin Qiao]

6 Zhaohai confluent Yin Qiao

2 Rangu [ying-spring]

9 Zhubin [xi-cleft Yin Wei]

7 Fuliu [jing-river]

3 Taixi [yuan, shu-stream]

4 Dazhong [luo]

5 Shuiquan [xi-cleft]

Figure 8.5 The Kidney Channel — Stage 5

THE KIDNEY CHANNEL — CASE STUDY

Mr HB, 38 year old married computer consultant with two children

Mr HB has been working long hours, getting home late and having difficulty going to sleep. He complains of recent profound fatigue, low back pain with no radiation, reduced libido and difficulties sustaining an erection. He has frequent small urinations, nocturia (1–2x/night), a daily soft bowel motion, pale complexion, dark shadows under both eyes, cold hands and feet, aching cold knees and poor tolerance to exercise (unable to play with the children after work). Recently he has been fearful of being made redundant at work.

QUESTIONS

Circle or write your answers as required.

1 Is this an external or internal disorder?

2 If external:

  (a) Is it due to heat or cold?

  (b) Are there symptoms of wind, dampness or dryness?

  (c) Is it acute, chronic or a mixed condition?

3 If internal:

  (a) Is it due to deficiency or excess?

   (i) If deficient, is it: qi, blood, jin ye, yin or yang?

   (ii) If excess, is it: stagnant qi, stagnant blood, damp/phlegm, rebellious qi, rising liver yang, empty fire etc?

  (b) Is it due to cold or heat?

  (c) Which zang fu are affected?

  (d) Which channels are affected?

4 **What might the pulse feel like?**
Describe: pulse rate, rhythm, depth, shape and strength.

5 **What might the tongue look like?**
Describe:
 – tongue body (colour, shape, thickness)
 – tongue coating (moisture, colour, thickness, distribution, root).

6 **What is the Chinese diagnosis?**
Where appropriate discuss the root (ben), the presenting symptoms (biao) and the five phase/ wu xing dynamics (the relationship between and among the zang fu organs under syndromes of imbalance or disease).

7 **What is your treatment principle?**

8 **What points would you use and why? Include adjunctive therapy such as moxa and cupping, if appropriate.**
(A minimum of five points, use only points on the Lung, Large Intestine, Stomach, Spleen, Heart, Small Intestine, Bladder and Kidney Channels.)

Chapter Nine

THE PERICARDIUM CHANNEL OF HAND JUEYIN

手厥阴心包经

The Pericardium Channel of Hand Jueyin is *biao li* partnered with the San jiao Channel and paired with the Liver Channel according to six channel theory.

The use of the Pericardium Channel is based on knowing the functions and indications of the Pericardium Channel points and the pathophysiology of the pericardium as a '*heart wrapper*'.

The Pericardium Channel connects with the following zang fu:

San Jiao

The main pathway:

- emerges 1 cun lateral to the nipple at Tianchi PC1
- arches over the axilla to Tianquan PC2, 2 cun below the anterior axillary fold
- descends to the anticubital fossa of the elbow between the Lung and Heart Channels
- continues down the forearm between the tendons of palmaris longus and flexor carpi radialis to reach the palm
- crosses the palm, travels down the middle finger and ends at the tip at Zhongchong PC9.

The other branches:

- two branches begin in the centre of the chest

- one branch connects with the pericardium and then descends through the diaphragm to the abdomen, connecting successively with the upper, middle and lower jiao (San Jiao)

- a second branch runs inside the chest and emerges in the costal region 3 cun below the anterior axillary fold 1 cun lateral to the nipple at Tianchi PC1 (see main pathway)

- another small connecting branch rises from the palm at Laogong PC8, and runs along the radial aspect of the ring finger to its tip where it links with the San Jiao Channel of Hand Shaoyang at Guanchong SJ1.

The Pericardium Channel has no connections with other primary channels at any points on the body.

THE PERICARDIUM CHANNEL POINTS			
WHO number	Pinyin	Name	Specific functions
PC1	**Tianchi**	Celestial Pool	
PC2	**Tianquan**	Celestial Spring	
PC3	**Quze**	Marsh at the Bend	He-Sea*5
PC4	**Ximen**	Cleft-Xi Gate	Xi-Cleft
PC5	**Jianshi**	Intermediary Courier	Jing-River*4
PC6	**Neiguan**	Inner Pass	Luo-Connecting, Confluent Yin Wei Mai
PC7	**Daling**	Great Mound	Yuan-Source, Shu-Stream*3
PC8	**Laogong**	Palace of Toil	Ying-Spring*2
PC9	**Zhongchong**	Central Hub	Jing-Well*1

* The 5 Shu points of the Yin Channels:
    1 = wood
    2 = fire
    3 = earth
    4 = metal
    5 = water

Note: The 9 points highlighted in bold are provided on the composite diagram for this channel (the fifth diagram).

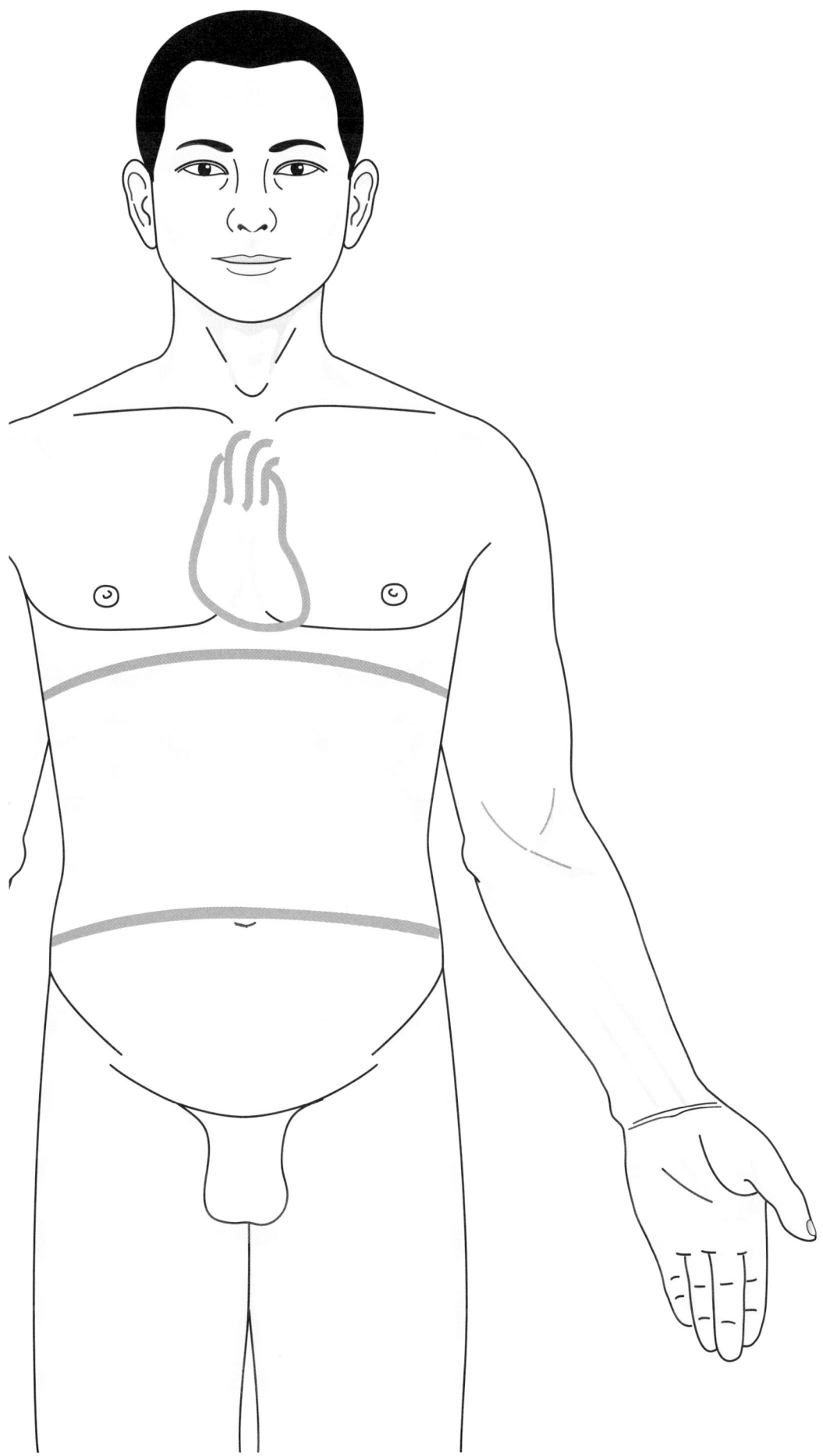

Figure 9.1 Pericardium Channel — Stage 1

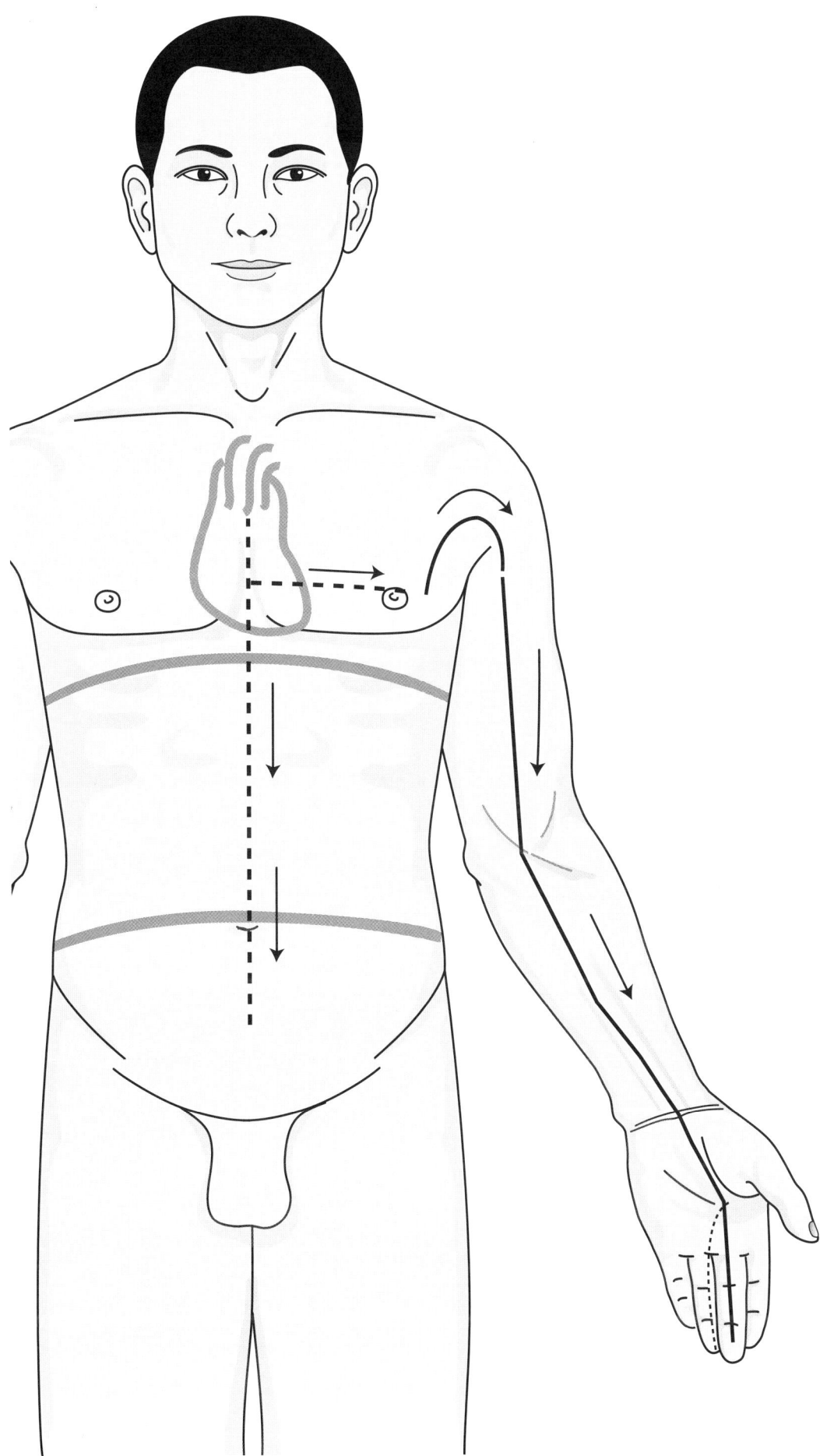

Figure 9.2 Pericardium Channel — Stage 2

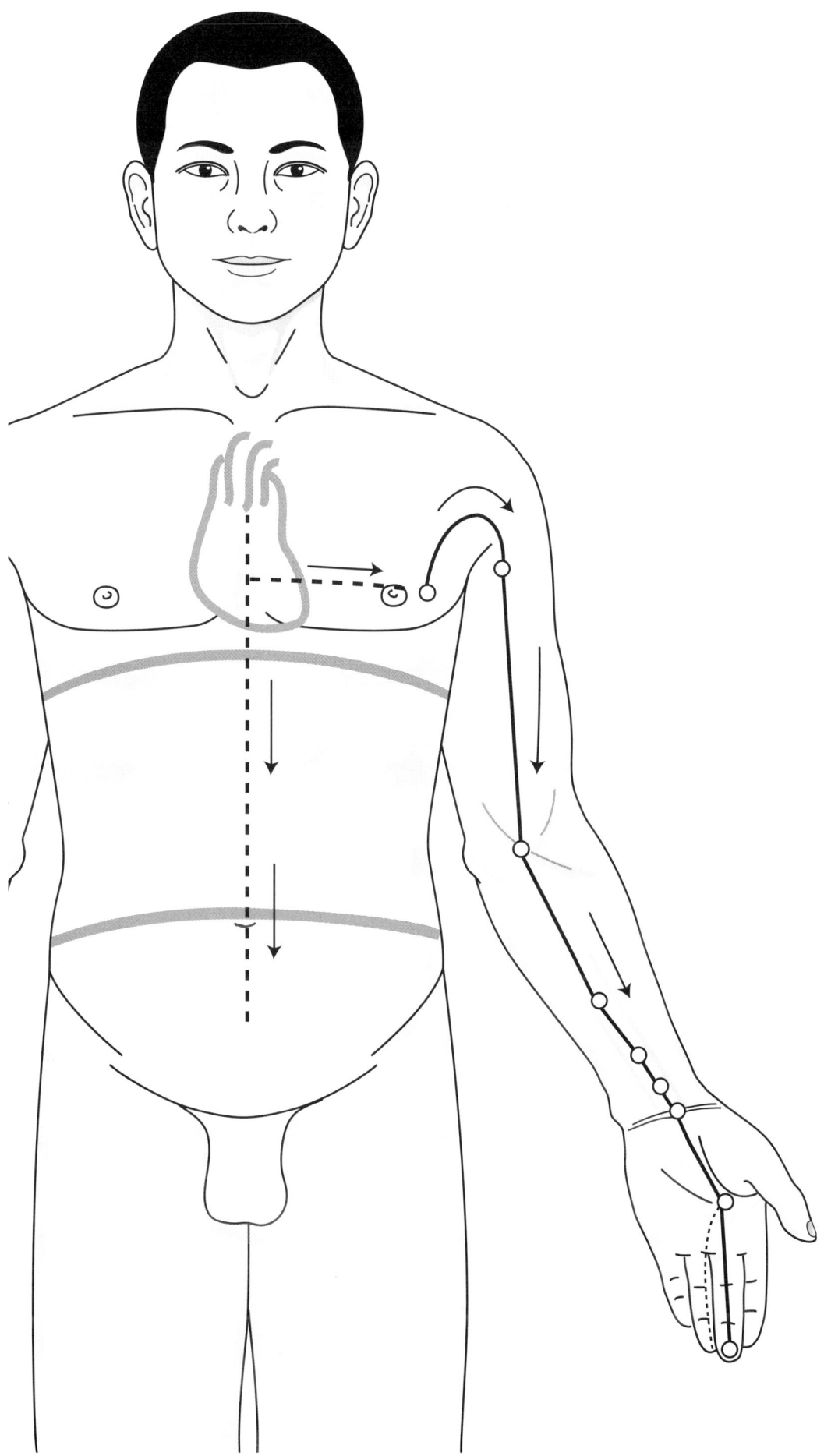

Figure 9.3 Pericardium Channel — Stage 3

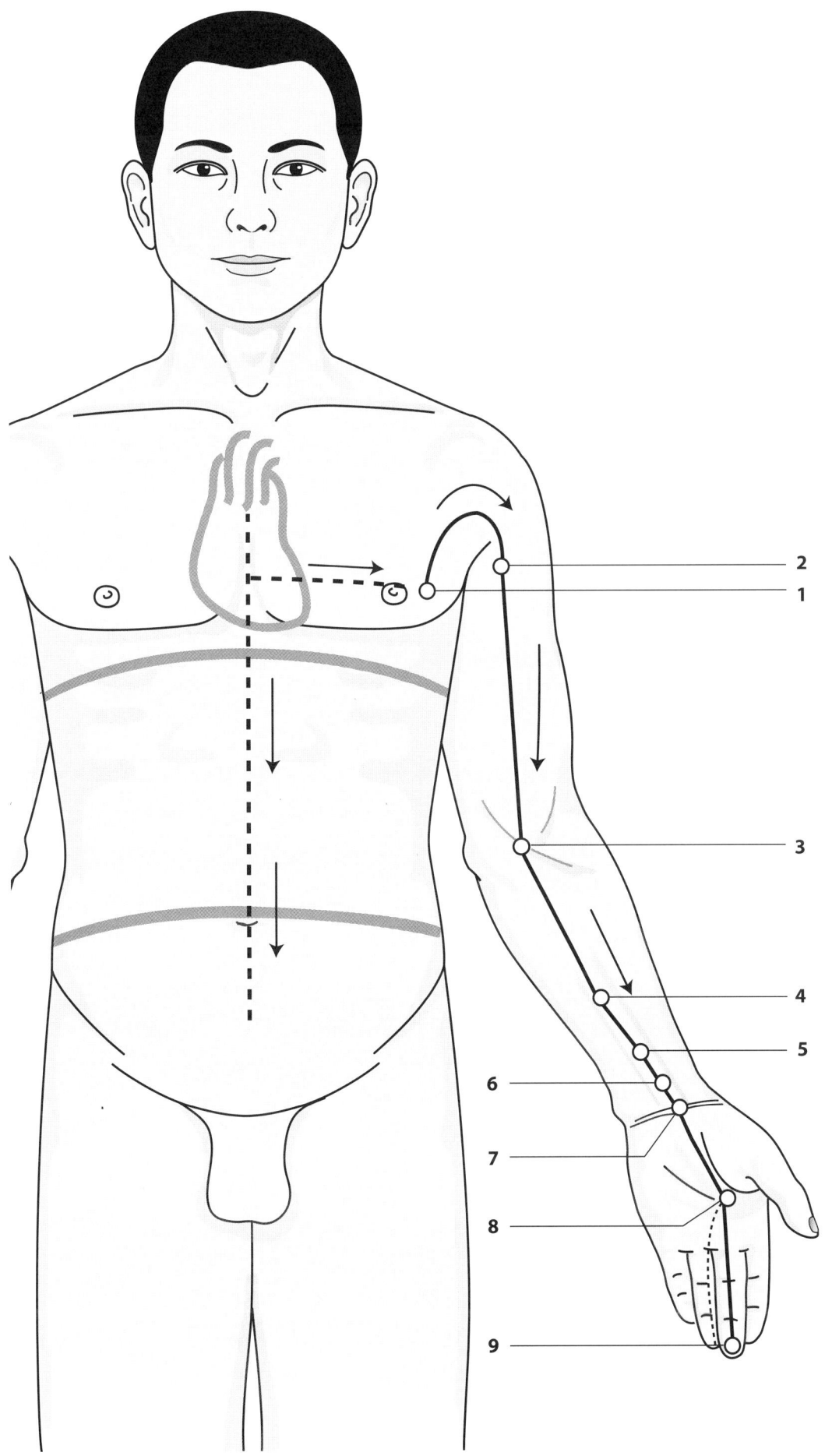

Figure 9.4 Pericardium Channel — Stage 4

yuan — blue	
luo — red	
xi-cleft — green	
five shu — yellow	
lower he-sea — orange	
back-shu — purple	

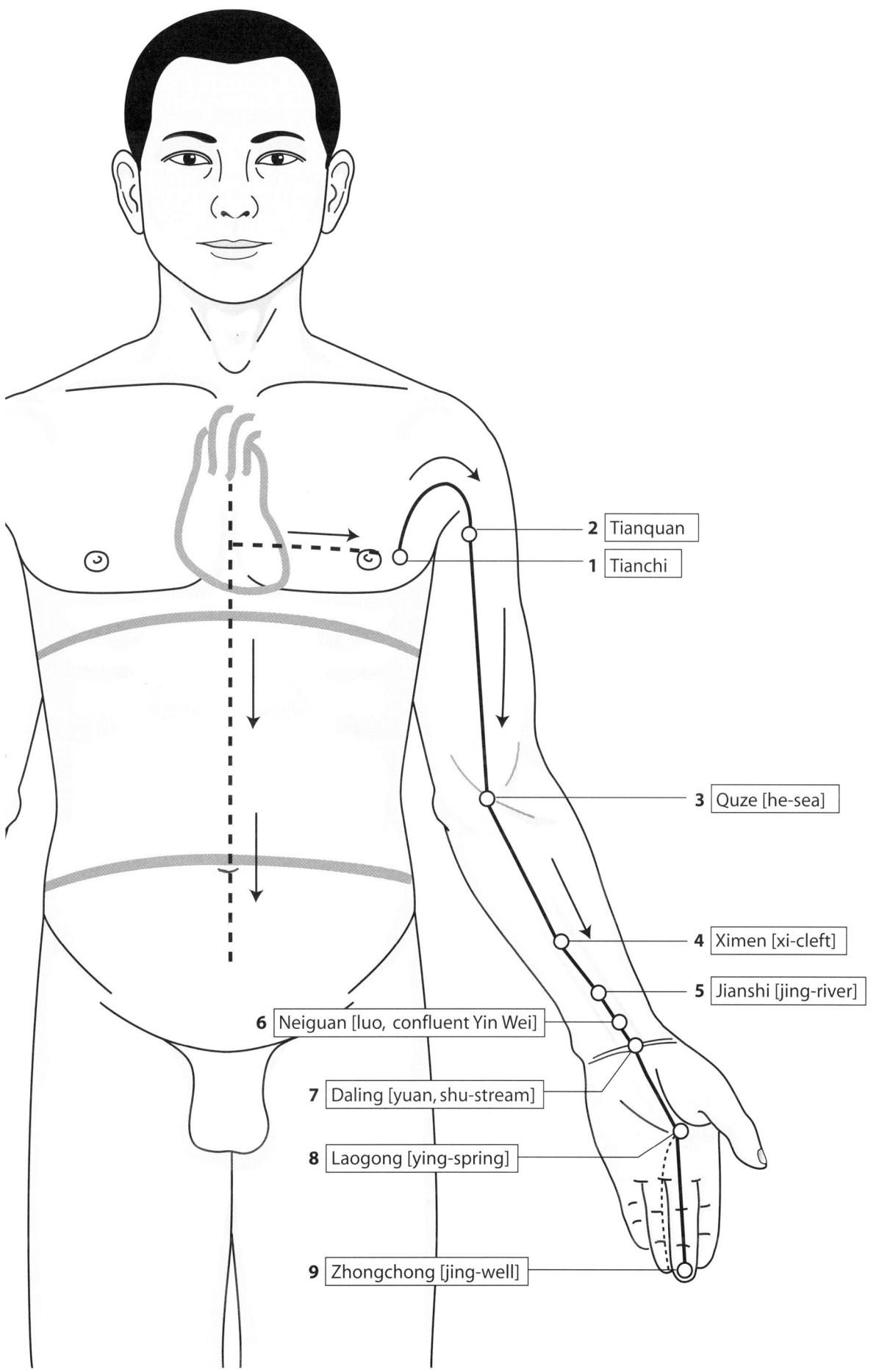

2 Tianquan
1 Tianchi
3 Quze [he-sea]
4 Ximen [xi-cleft]
5 Jianshi [jing-river]
6 Neiguan [luo, confluent Yin Wei]
7 Daling [yuan, shu-stream]
8 Laogong [ying-spring]
9 Zhongchong [jing-well]

Figure 9.5 Pericardium Channel — Stage 5

THE PERICARDIUM CHANNEL — CASE STUDY

Mr CB, 46 year old warehouse manager

Mr CB presents with acute stabbing pain in the heart region which radiates to the shoulder, down the left arm and up into the neck. He has used a coronary artery vasodilator spray and the pain is now subsiding. He complains of shortness of breath, a sense of heaviness and restriction in the chest, cold hands and feet, and is restless and worried. His complexion is pale, and his lips and fingernails are 'blue'. A previous ECG diagnosed angina.

QUESTIONS

Circle or write your answers as required.

1 Is this an external or internal disorder?

2 If external:
   (a) Is it due to heat or cold?

   (b) Are there symptoms of wind, dampness or dryness?

   (c) Is it acute, chronic or a mixed condition?

3 If internal:
   (a) Is it due to deficiency or excess?

      (i)   If deficient, is it: qi, blood, jin ye, yin or yang?

      (ii) If excess, is it: stagnant qi, stagnant blood, damp/phlegm, rebellious qi, rising liver yang, empty fire etc?

   (b) Is it due to cold or heat?

   (c) Which zang fu are affected?

   (d) Which channels are affected?

4 **What might the pulse feel like?**
Describe: pulse rate, rhythm, depth, shape and strength.

5 **What might the tongue look like?**
Describe:
  – tongue body (colour, shape, thickness)
  – tongue coating (moisture, colour, thickness, distribution, root).

6 **What is the Chinese diagnosis?**
Where appropriate discuss the root (ben), the presenting symptoms (biao) and the five phase/ wu xing dynamics (the relationship between and among the zang fu organs under syndromes of imbalance or disease).

7 **What is your treatment principle?**

8 **What points would you use and why? Include adjunctive therapy such as moxa or cupping if appropriate.**
(A minimum of five points, use only points on the Lung, Large Intestine, Stomach, Spleen, Heart, Small Intestine, Bladder, Kidney and Pericardium Channels.)

Chapter Ten

THE SAN JIAO CHANNEL OF HAND SHAOYANG

手少阳三焦经

The San Jiao Channel of Hand Shaoyang is *biao li* partnered with the Pericardium Channel and paired with the Gall Bladder Channel according to six channel theory.

The use of the San Jiao Channel is based on knowing the functions and indications of the San jiao Channel points and the pathophysiology of the San Jiao as a *fu*.

The San Jiao Channel connects with the following zang fu:

San Jiao (upper, middle & lower)   Pericardium

The main pathway:

- begins at the ulnar aspect of the tip of the ring finger at Guanchong SJ1

- runs upward between the fourth and fifth metacarpal bones along the dorsal aspect of the hand and wrist

- travels up the forearm between the radius and ulna and between the Large and Small Intestine Channels

- passes over the olecranon and continues along the lateral aspect of the upper arm to the posterior aspect of the shoulder

- travels medially towards the spine intersecting with the Small Intestine Channel and Du Mai

- ascends laterally to Jianjing GB21 and descends into the supraclavicular fossa (see other branches)

- the chest branch emerges from the supraclavicular fossa and runs upward along the neck to the posterior border of the ear

- circles up and around behind the ear to Jiaosun SJ20 (see other branches)

- an auricular branch separates behind the ear in the region of Yifeng GB17, enters the ear and then emerges in front of the ear

- crosses the temple and the descending branch, to reach the outer end of the eyebrow on the supraorbital rim at Sizhukong SJ23, where it links with the Gall Bladder Channel of Foot Shaoyang at Tongziliao GB1.

The other branches:

- a branch descends from the supraclavicular fossa, disperses midway between the breasts, connects with the pericardium, then descends through the diaphragm, linking along its pathway with the upper, middle and lower jiao

- another branch separates from the chest in the region of Shanzhong Ren17, running upward where it emerges from the supraclavicular fossa and continues as the main pathway (see above)

- from Jiaosun SJ20, a branch crosses the temple and ascends to the anterior hairline where it turns and runs downward through the cheek, then turns and ascends to the inferior aspect of the eye

- according to the Spiritual Pivot, a branch descends from the lower jiao to Weiyang BL39.

The San Jiao Channel connects with other primary channels at various points on the body, specifically the Small Intestine, Bladder, Du Mai, Gall Bladder, Stomach and Ren Mai Channels.

THE SAN JIAO CHANNEL POINTS

WHO number	Pinyin	Name	Specific functions
SJ1	**Guanchong**	Passage Hub	Jing-Well*1
SJ2	**Yemen**	Fluid (*humour*) Gate	Ying-Spring*2
SJ3	**Zhongzhu**	Central Islet	Shu-Stream*3
SJ4	**Yangchi**	Yang Pool	Yuan-Source
SJ5	**Waiguan**	Outer Pass	Luo-Connecting, Confluent Yang Wei Mai
SJ6	**Zhigou**	Branch Ditch	Jing-River*4
SJ7	**Huizong**	Convergence & Gathering	Xi-Cleft
SJ8	**Sanyangluo**	Three Yang Connection	
SJ9	**Sidu**	Four Rivers	
SJ10	**Tianjing**	Celestial Well	He-Sea*5
SJ11	Qinglengyuan	Clear Cold Abyss	
SJ12	Xiaoluo	Dispersing Riverbed	
SJ13	**Naohui**	Upper Arm Convergence	
SJ14	**Jianliao**	Shoulder Bone-Hole	
SJ15	**Tianliao**	Celestial Bone-Hole	
SJ16	**Tianyou**	Celestial Window	
SJ17	**Yifeng**	Wind Screen	
SJ18	Qimai	Spasm Vessel	
SJ19	Luxi	Skull Rest	
SJ20	**Jiaosun**	Angle Vertex	
SJ21	**Ermen**	Ear Gate	
SJ22	Erheliao	Harmony Bone-Hole	
SJ23	**Sizhukong**	Silk Bamboo Hole	

* The 5 Shu points of the Yang Channels:
   1 = metal
   2 = water
   3 = wood
   4 = fire
   5 = earth

Note: The 18 points highlighted in bold are provided on the composite diagram for this channel (the fifth diagram).

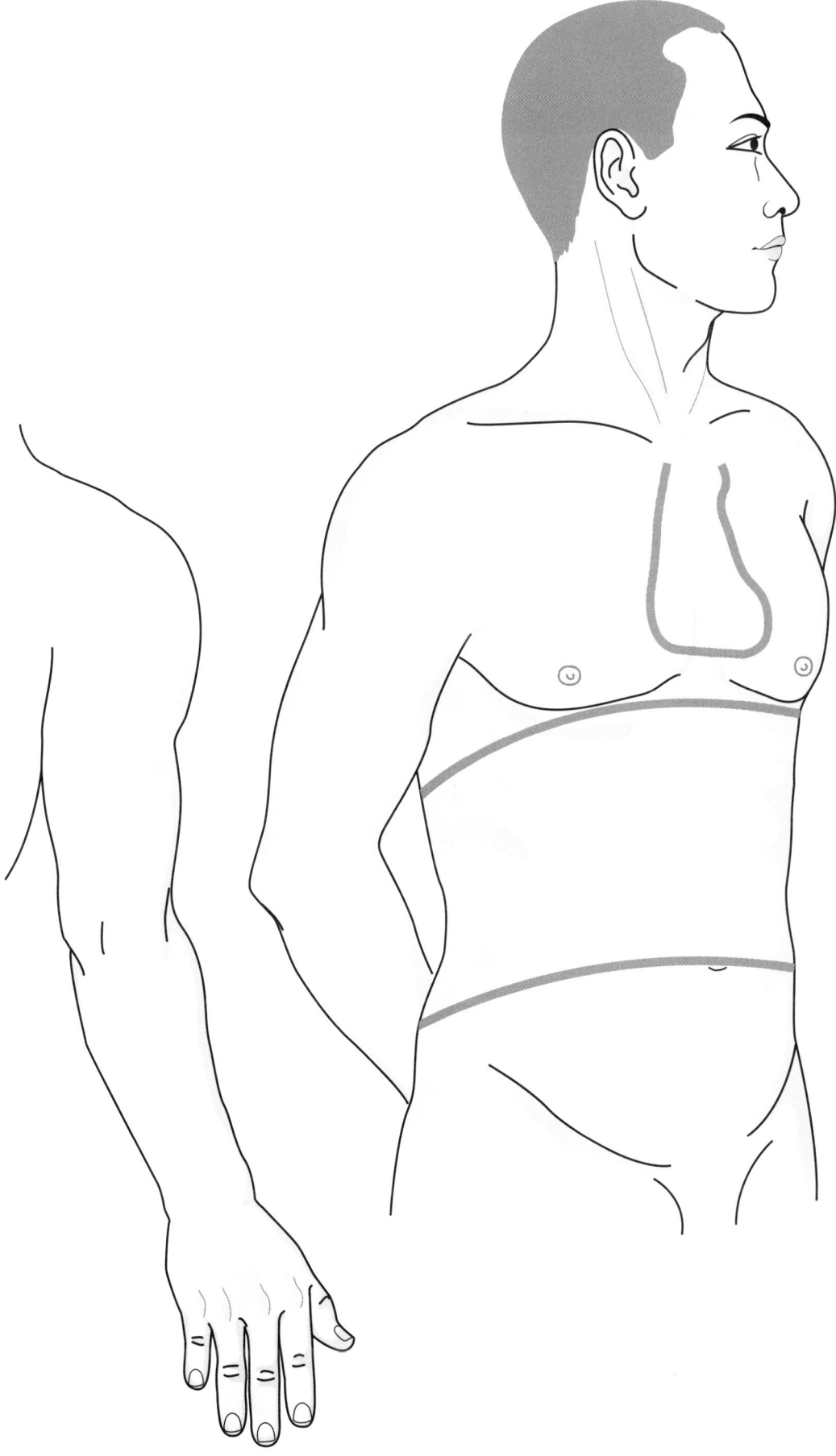

Figure 10.1 San Jiao Channel — Stage 1

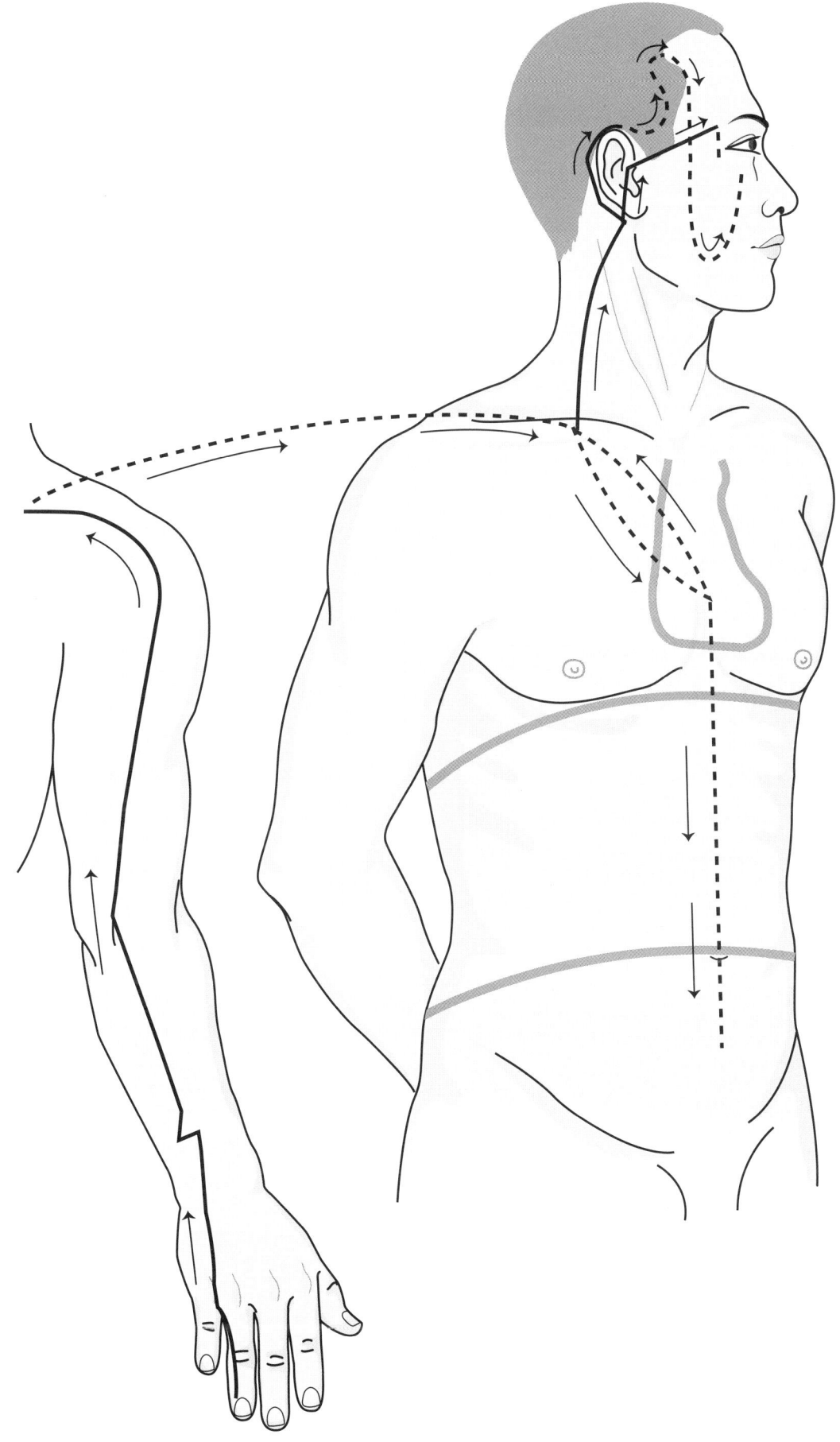

Figure 10.2 San Jiao Channel — Stage 2

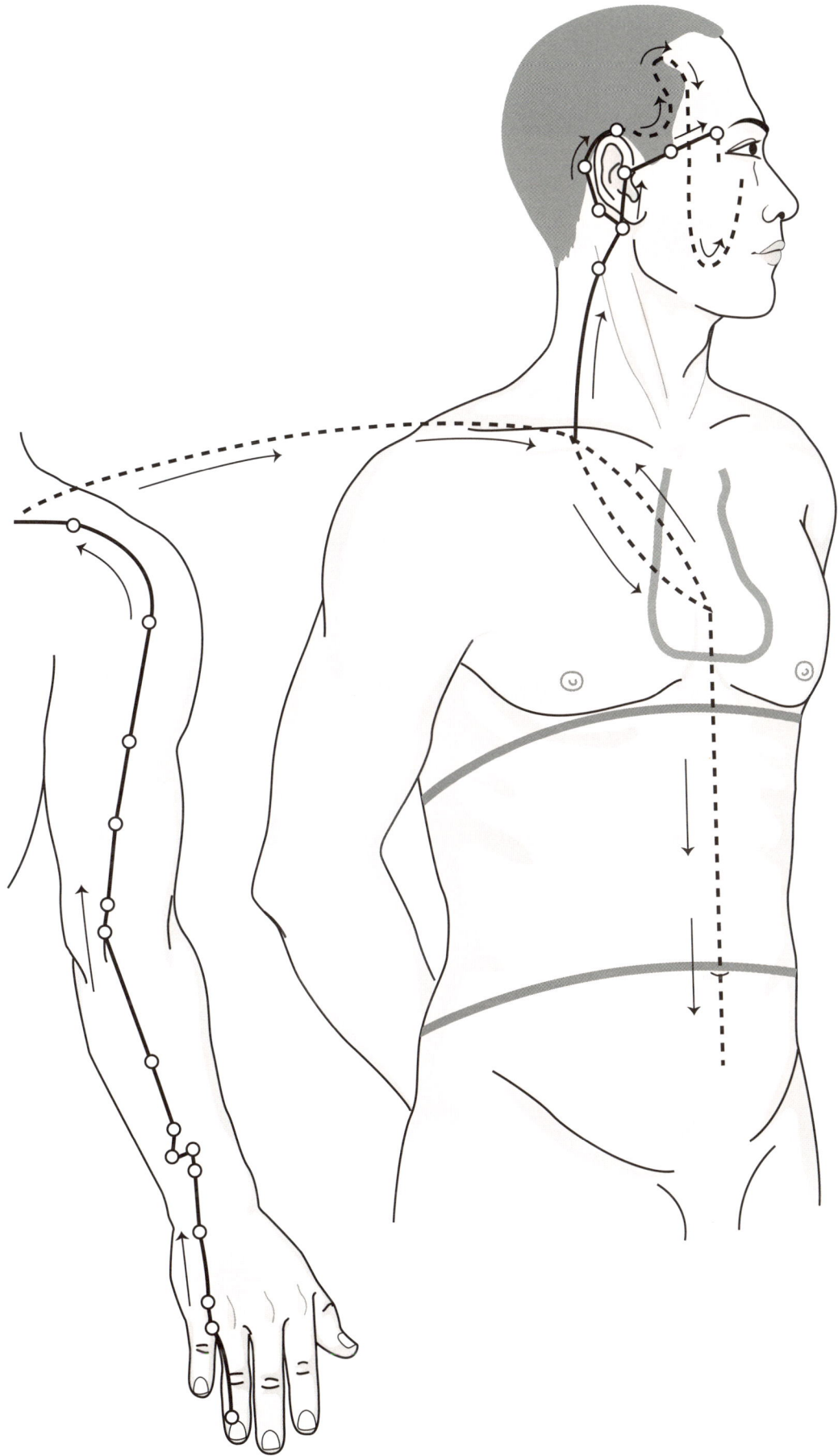

Figure 10.3 San Jiao Channel — Stage 3

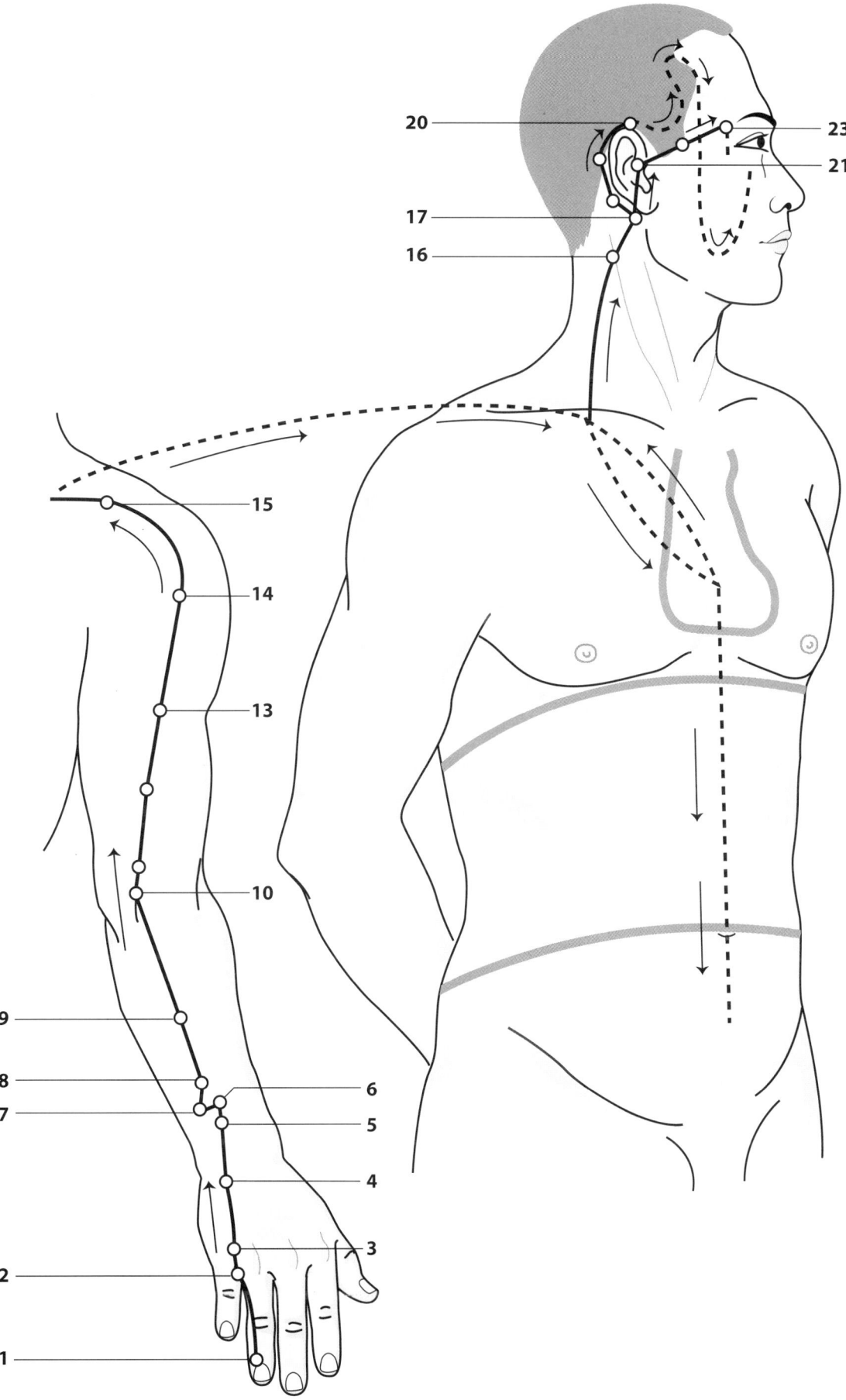

Figure 10.4 San Jiao Channel — Stage 4

| yuan — blue |
| luo — red |
| xi-cleft — green |
| five shu — yellow |
| lower he-sea — orange |
| back-shu — purple |

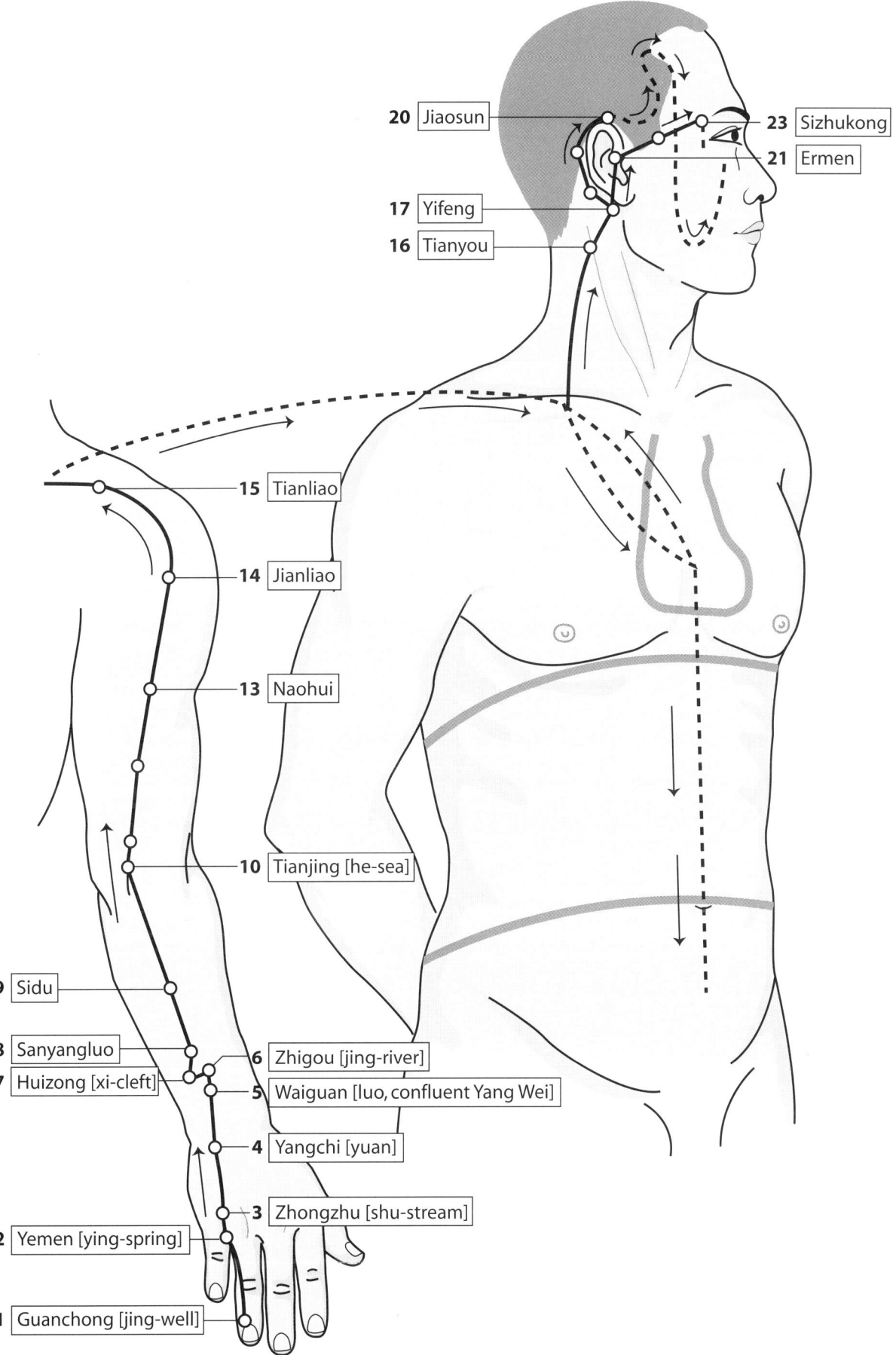

20 Jiaosun

23 Sizhukong

21 Ermen

17 Yifeng

16 Tianyou

15 Tianliao

14 Jianliao

13 Naohui

10 Tianjing [he-sea]

9 Sidu

8 Sanyangluo

7 Huizong [xi-cleft]

6 Zhigou [jing-river]

5 Waiguan [luo, confluent Yang Wei]

4 Yangchi [yuan]

3 Zhongzhu [shu-stream]

2 Yemen [ying-spring]

1 Guanchong [jing-well]

Figure 10.5 San Jiao Channel — Stage 5

THE SAN JIAO CHANNEL — CASE STUDY

Mrs JC, 70 year old pensioner who lives alone

Mrs JC is a fit, independent healthy pensioner with no current medical problems. She is a non-smoker, takes some nutritional supplements and is not on any Western medication. Recently she fell and injured her right wrist and forearm. She complains of restricted hand and wrist movements, heat and swelling of the forearm and wrist, and difficulty with normal activities such as cooking, gardening and writing.

QUESTIONS

Circle or write your answers as required.

1 Is this an external or internal disorder?

2 If external:

(a) Is it due to heat or cold?

(b) Are there symptoms of wind, dampness or dryness?

(c) Is it acute, chronic or a mixed condition?

3 If internal:

(a) Is it due to deficiency or excess?

(i) If deficient, is it: qi, blood, jin ye, yin or yang?

(ii) If excess, is it: stagnant qi, stagnant blood, damp/phlegm, rebellious qi, rising liver yang, empty fire etc?

(b) Is it due to cold or heat?

(c) Which zang fu are affected?

(d) Which channels are affected?

4 **What might the pulse feel like?**
    Describe: pulse rate, rhythm, depth, shape and strength.

5 **What might the tongue look like?**
    Describe:
    – tongue body (colour, shape, thickness)
    – tongue coating (moisture, colour, thickness, distribution, root).

6 **What is the Chinese diagnosis?**
    Where appropriate discuss the root (ben), the presenting symptoms (biao) and the five phase/ wu xing dynamics (the relationship between and among the zang fu organs under syndromes of imbalance or disease).

7 **What is your treatment principle?**

8 **What points would you use and why? Include adjunctive therapy such as moxa or cupping if appropriate.**
    (A minimum of five points, use only points on the Lung, Large Intestine, Stomach, Spleen, Heart, Small Intestine, Bladder, Kidney, Pericardium and San jiao Channels.)

Chapter Eleven

THE GALL BLADDER CHANNEL OF FOOT SHAOYANG

足少阳胆经

The Gall Bladder Channel of Foot Shaoyang is *biao li* partnered with the Liver Channel and paired with the San jiao Channel according to six channel theory.

The use of the Gall Bladder Channel is based on knowing the functions and indications of the Gall Bladder Channel points and the pathophysiology of the gall bladder as an extraordinary *fu*.

The Gall Bladder Channel connects with the following zang fu:

Gall Bladder   Liver

The main pathway:

- starts near the outer canthus of the eye at Tongziliao GB1 (see other branches)

- crosses the cheek to Tinghui GB2 anterior to the intertragic notch

- ascends over the zygomatic arch and runs upward within the anterior hairline of the temporal region to Hanyan GB4

- curves posteriorly and runs around the ear outside the San Jiao line to Wangu GB12 at the mastoid process

- from there it turns back and curves up around the side of the head to the corner of the forehead at Touwei ST8 and then descends to the supraorbital region at Yangbai GB14

- it then ascends and curves back across the top of the head descending to Fengchi GB20, just below the occiput

- continues down the neck and out to the high point of the shoulder at Jianjing GB21 (see other branches)

- a branch continues downward from the supraclavicular fossa and passes in front of the axilla along the lateral aspect of the chest

- passes down through the free ends of the floating ribs (lower border of 11th and 12th ribs) to the hip joint where it meets the internal branch arising from the outer canthus

- descends along the lateral aspect of the thigh and through the lateral side of the knee
- continues downward along the anterior aspect of the fibula until it reaches the anterior aspect of the lateral malleolus
- follows the dorsal surface of the foot along the groove between the fourth and fifth metatarsals, to end on the lateral side of the tip of the fourth toenail at Zuqiaoyin GB44.

The other branches:

- a branch rises from Jianjing GB21 to meet with the spine at Dazhui Du14, passes laterally to Bingfeng SI12, then descends anteriorly into the supraclavicular fossa (see main pathway)
- the auricular branch rises from behind the ear, enters the ear at Yifeng SJ17, emerges in front of the ear and passes via Tinggong SI19 and Xiaguan ST7, to the posterior aspect of the outer canthus
- another branch rising from the outer canthus runs down to the corner of the jaw at Daying ST5, loops around and up to meet the San Jiao Channel in the infraorbital region, passes back down through Jiache ST6, runs down the neck and enters the supraclavicular fossa where it meets the main channel
- from here it descends into the chest, passes through the diaphragm, connects with the liver and gall bladder, continues along the inside of the ribs to emerge in the inguinal region near the femoral artery, runs superficially inside the upper border of the pubic hair, enters deeply into the sacral region and emerges on the buttock at Huantiao GB30
- the foot branch springs from Zulingqi GB41, runs between the first and second metatarsal toes to the distal portion of the big toe, where it links with the Liver Channel of Foot Jueyin.

The Gall Bladder Channel connects with other primary channels at various points on the body, specifically the Stomach, Small Intestine, Bladder, Pericardium, San Jiao, Liver and Du Mai Channels.

THE GALL BLADDER CHANNEL POINTS

WHO number	Pinyin	Name	Specific functions
GB1	**Tongziliao**	Pupil Bone-Hole	
GB2	**Tinghui**	Auditory Convergence	
GB3	**Shangguan**	Upper Gate	
GB4	**Hanyan**	Forehead Fullness	
GB5	**Xuanlu**	Suspended Skull	
GB6	Xuanli	Suspended Tuft	
GB7	Qubin	Temporal Hairline Curve	
GB8	**Shuaigu**	Valley Lead	
GB9	Tianchong	Celestial Hub	
GB10	Fubai	Floating White	
GB11	Touqiaoyin	Head Portal Yin	
GB12	**Wangu**	Mastoid Process	
GB13	Benshen	Root Spirit	
GB14	**Yangbai**	Yang White	
GB15	Toulinqi	Head Overlooking Tears	
GB16	Muchuang	Eye Window	
GB17	Zhengying	Upright Construction	
GB18	Chengling	Spirit Support	
GB19	Naokong	Brain Hollow	
GB20	**Fengchi**	Wind Pool	

WHO number	Pinyin	Name	Specific functions
GB21	**Jianjing**	Shoulder Well	
GB22	Yuanye	Armpit Abyss	
GB23	Zhejin	Sinew Seat	
GB24	**Riyue**	Sun and Moon	Front-Mu (GB)
GB25	**Jingmen**	Capital Gate	Front-Mu (KI)
GB26	**Daimai**	Girdling Vessel	
GB27	**Wushu**	Fifth Pivot	
GB28	**Weidao**	Linking Path	
GB29	**Juliao**	Squatting Bone-Hole	
GB30	**Huantiao**	Jumping Round	
GB31	**Fengshi**	Wind Market	
GB32	Zhongdu	Central River	
GB33	Xiyangguan	Knee Yang Joint	
GB34	**Yanglingquan**	Yang Mound Spring	Influential Point of Tendon, He-Sea*5
GB35	**Yangjiao**	Yang Intersection	Xi-Cleft Yang Wei Mai
GB36	**Waiqiu**	Outer Hill	Xi-Cleft
GB37	**Guangming**	Bright Light	Luo-Connecting
GB38	**Yangfu**	Yang Assistance	Jing-River*4
GB39	**Xuanzhong**	Suspended Bell	Influential Point of Marrow
GB40	**Qiuxu**	Hill Ruins	Yuan-Source
GB41	**Zulingqi**	Foot Overlooking Tears	Confluent Dai Mai, Shu-Stream*3
GB42	Diwuhui	Earth Fivefold Convergence	
GB43	**Xiaxi**	Pinched Ravine	Ying-Spring*2
GB44	**Zuqiaoyin**	Foot Portal Yin	Jing-Well*1

* The 5 Shu points of the Yang Channels:
      1 = metal
      2 = water
      3 = wood
      4 = fire
      5 = earth

Note: The 28 points highlighted in bold are provided on the composite diagram for this channel (the fifth diagram).

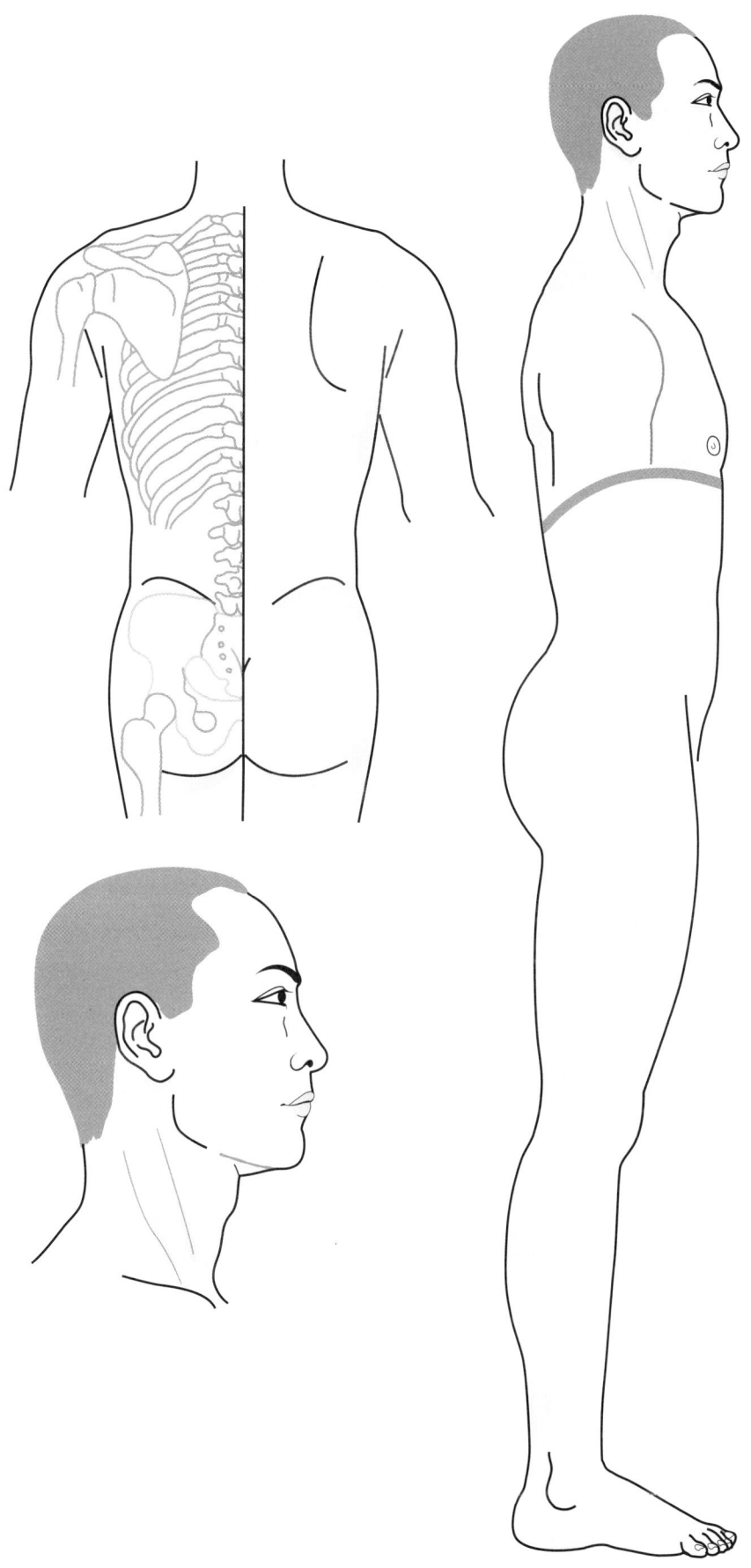

Figure 11.1 Gall Bladder Channel — Stage 1

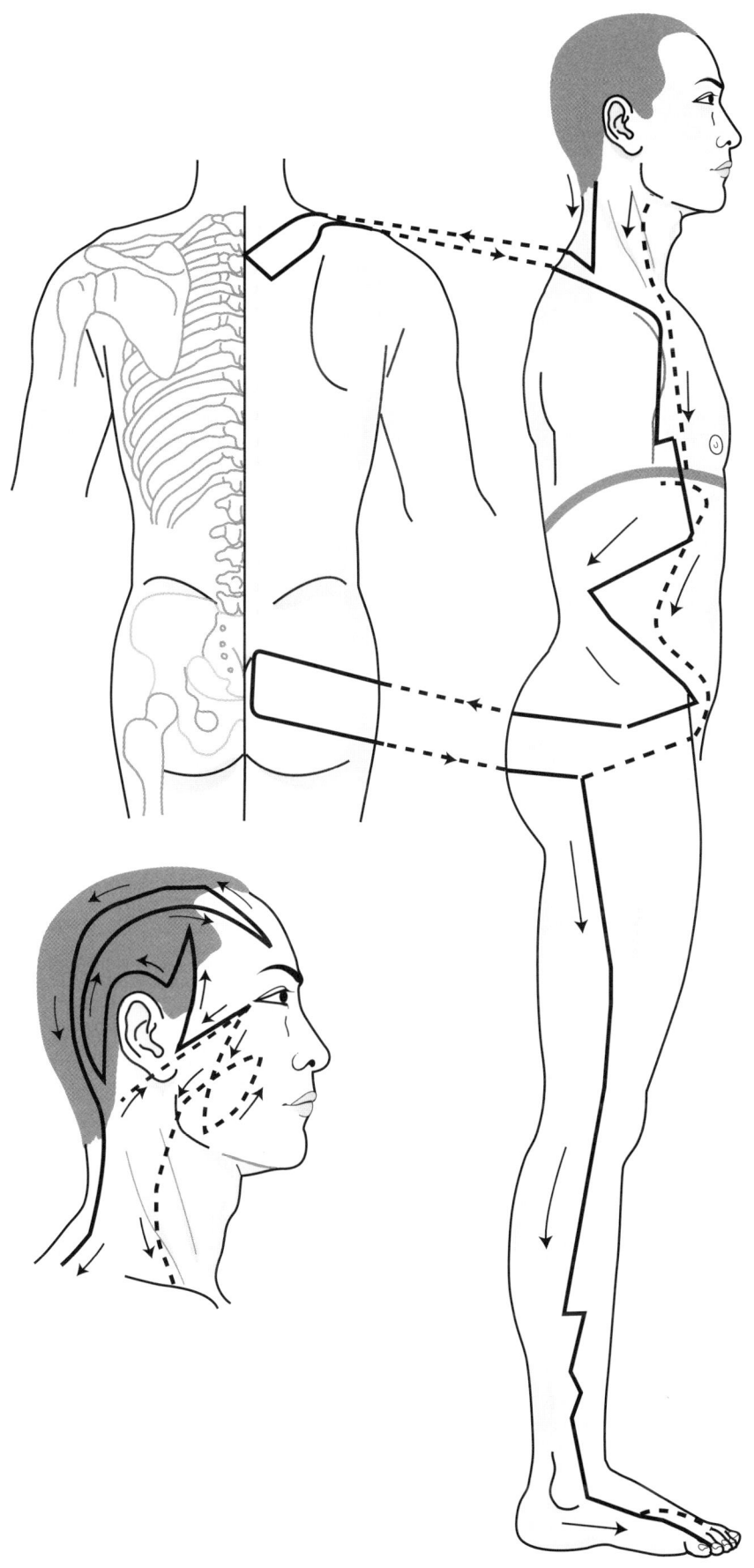

Figure 11.2 Gall Bladder Channel — Stage 2

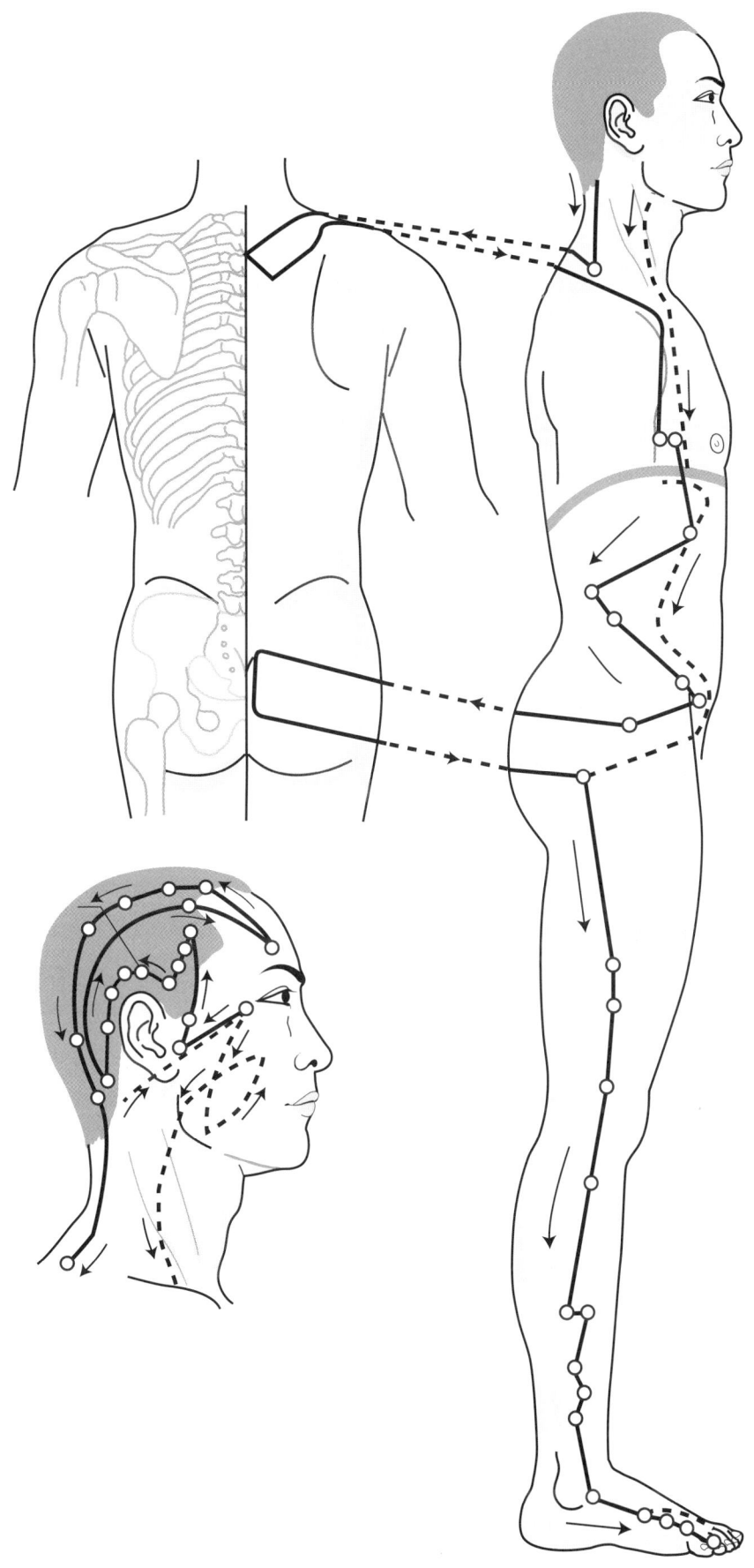

Figure 11.3 Gall Bladder Channel — Stage 3

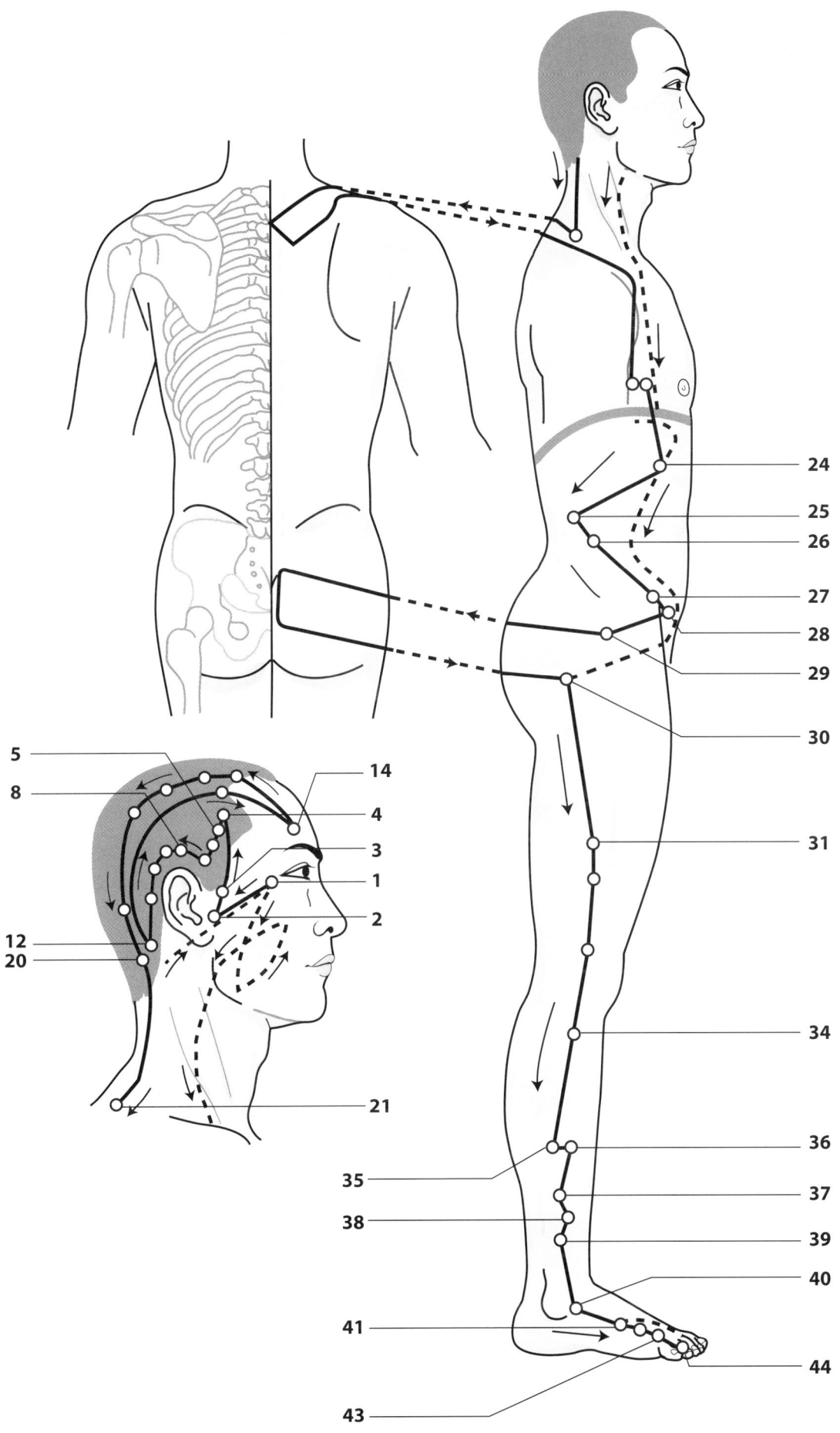

Figure 11.4 Gall Bladder Channel — Stage 4

yuan — blue
luo — red
xi-cleft — green
five shu — yellow
lower he-sea — orange
back-shu — purple

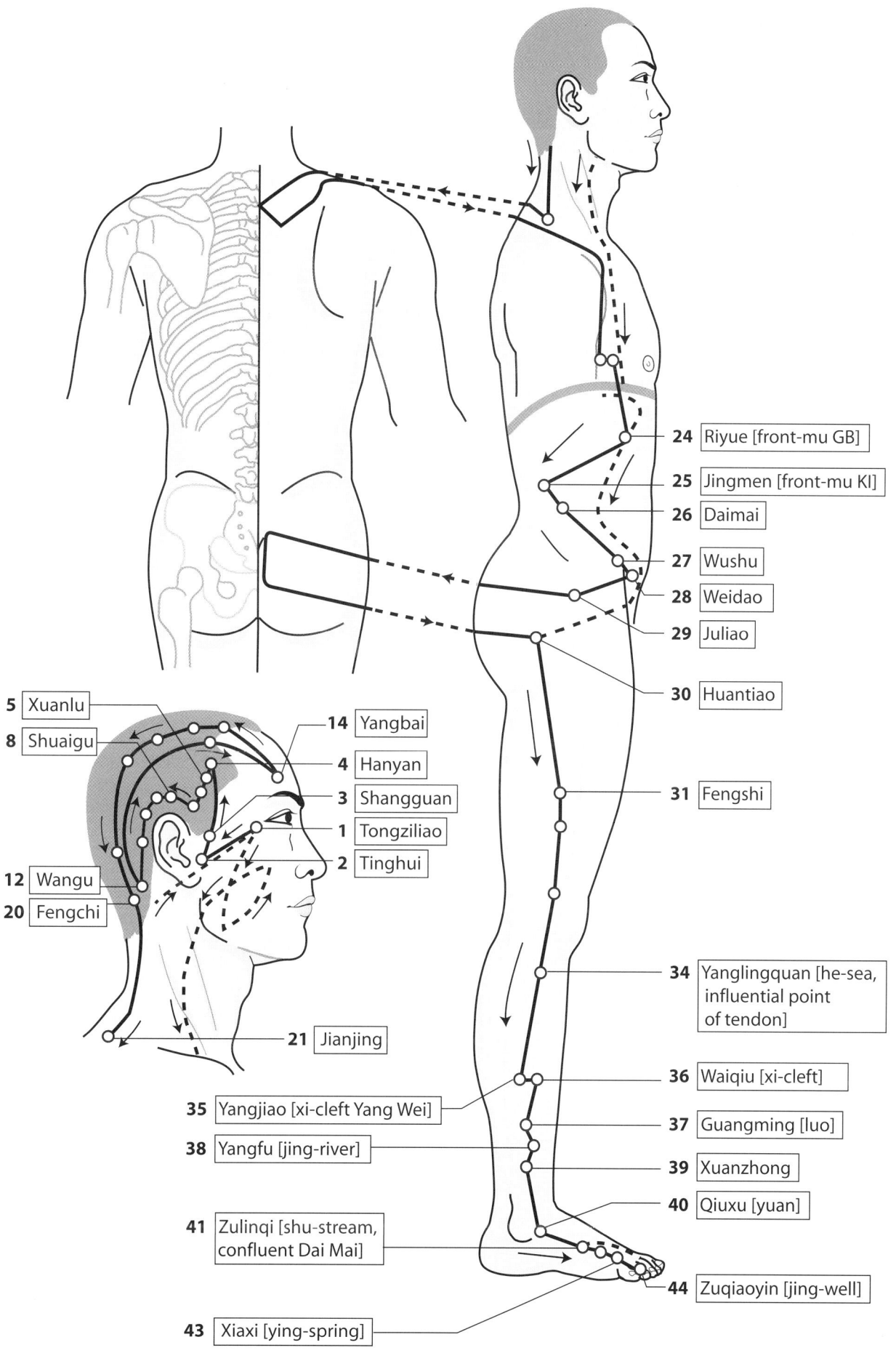

24 Riyue [front-mu GB]

25 Jingmen [front-mu KI]

26 Daimai

27 Wushu

28 Weidao

29 Juliao

30 Huantiao

31 Fengshi

5 Xuanlu

8 Shuaigu

14 Yangbai

4 Hanyan

3 Shangguan

1 Tongziliao

2 Tinghui

12 Wangu

20 Fengchi

21 Jianjing

34 Yanglingquan [he-sea, influential point of tendon]

35 Yangjiao [xi-cleft Yang Wei]

38 Yangfu [jing-river]

36 Waiqiu [xi-cleft]

37 Guangming [luo]

39 Xuanzhong

40 Qiuxu [yuan]

41 Zulinqi [shu-stream, confluent Dai Mai]

44 Zuqiaoyin [jing-well]

43 Xiaxi [ying-spring]

Figure 11.5 Gall Bladder Channel — Stage 5

THE GALL BLADDER CHANNEL — CASE STUDY

Ms AB, 28 year old international flight attendant, Asia region

Ms AB has been feeling tired and below par for several weeks after returning from Asia. Friends say she 'looks yellow' (sallow). She complains of poor appetite, bloating, nausea, intolerance to fatty foods, sour taste in her mouth, thirst, colicky abdominal pain after meals, loose bowel motions and offensive flatus, and scanty dark-yellow urine. She is sore underneath her right rib cage. An ultrasound scan shows small stones in her gall bladder.

QUESTIONS

Circle or write your answers as required.

1   Is this an external or internal disorder?

2   If external:

(a) Is it due to heat or cold?

(b) Are there symptoms of wind, dampness or dryness?

(c) Is it acute, chronic or a mixed condition?

3   If internal:

(a) Is it due to deficiency or excess?

(i) If deficient, is it: qi, blood, jin ye, yin or yang?

(ii) If excess, is it: stagnant qi, stagnant blood, damp/phlegm, rebellious qi, rising liver yang, empty fire etc?

(b) Is it due to cold or heat?

(c) Which zang fu are affected?

(d) Which channels are affected?

4 **What might the pulse feel like?**
  Describe: pulse rate, rhythm, depth, shape and strength.

5 **What might the tongue look like?**
  Describe:
  – tongue body (colour, shape, thickness)
  – tongue coating (moisture, colour, thickness, distribution, root).

6 **What is the Chinese diagnosis?**
  Where appropriate discuss the root (ben), the presenting symptoms (biao) and the five phase/ wu xing dynamics (the relationship between and among the zang fu organs under syndromes of imbalance or disease).

7 **What is your treatment principle?**

8 **What points would you use and why? Include adjunctive therapy such as moxa or cupping if appropriate.**
  (A minimum of five points, use only points on the Lung, Large Intestine, Stomach, Spleen, Heart, Small Intestine, Bladder, Kidney, Pericardium, San jiao and Gall Bladder Channels.)

Chapter Twelve

THE LIVER CHANNEL OF FOOT JUEYIN

足厥阴肝经

The Liver Channel of Foot Jueyin is *biao li* partnered with the Gall Bladder Channel and paired with the Pericardium Channel according to six channel theory.

The use of the Liver Channel is based on knowing the functions and indications of the Liver Channel points and the pathophysiology of the liver as a *zang*.

The Liver Channel connects with the following zang fu:

Liver   Gall Bladder   Lung   Stomach

The main pathway:

- originates from the hairy dorsal region of the big toe at Dadun LR1

- runs along the dorsum of the foot, passing anterior to the medial malleolus

- intersects the Spleen Channel at Sanyinjiao SP6, then ascends along the medial aspect of the lower leg, anterior to the Spleen Channel, to an area 8 cun above the medial malleolus

- crosses and continues posterior to the Spleen Channel up to the knee

- runs upward along the medial aspect of the thigh to the pubic region where it encircles the genitals and ascends to enter the lower abdomen where it intersects with Ren Mai (see other branches)

- it then continues upward from the pubic region to finish in the sixth intercostal space, 4 cun lateral to the midline at Qimen LR14.

The other branches:

- a branch arises from the lower abdomen, ascends to curve around the stomach before entering the liver and gall bladder, continues up through the diaphragm, spreads out in the costal and hypochondriac regions, continues upward along the posterior aspect of the throat to the naso–pharynx where it links with the tissues surrounding the eye ('eye system'), and then runs up over the forehead to the vertex where it intersects with Du Mai at Baihui Du20

- another branch arises from the 'eye system', runs downward into the cheek and encircles the inner surface of the lips

- a third branch separates from the liver, passes through the diaphragm, runs into the lung where it links with the Lung Channel of Hand Taiyin and meets with Tianchi PC1.

The Liver Channel connects with other primary channels at various points on the body, specifically the Spleen, Ren Mai, Pericardium and Du Mai Channels.

THE LIVER CHANNEL POINTS

WHO number	Pinyin	Name	Specific functions
LR1	**Dadun**	Large Pile	Jing-Well*1
LR2	**Xingjian**	Moving Between	Ying-Spring*2
LR3	**Taichong**	Great Surge	Yuan-Source, Shu-Stream*3
LR4	**Zhongfeng**	Mound Centre	Jing-River*4
LR5	**Ligou**	Woodworm Canal	Luo-Connecting
LR6	**Zhongdu**	Central Metropolis	Xi-Cleft
LR7	**Xiguan**	Knee Joint	
LR8	**Ququan**	Spring at the Bend	He-Sea*5
LR9	Yinbao	Yin Bladder	
LR10	Zuwuli	Foot Five Li	
LR11	Yinlian	Yin Corner	
LR12	**Jimai**	Urgent Pulse	
LR13	**Zhangmen**	Camphorwood Gate	Front-Mu (SP), Influential Point of Zang Organs
LR14	**Qimen**	Cycle Gate	Front-Mu (LR)

* The 5 Shu points of the Yin Channels:
  1 = wood
  2 = fire
  3 = earth
  4 = metal
  5 = water

Note: The 11 points highlighted in bold are provided on the composite diagram for this channel (the fifth diagram).

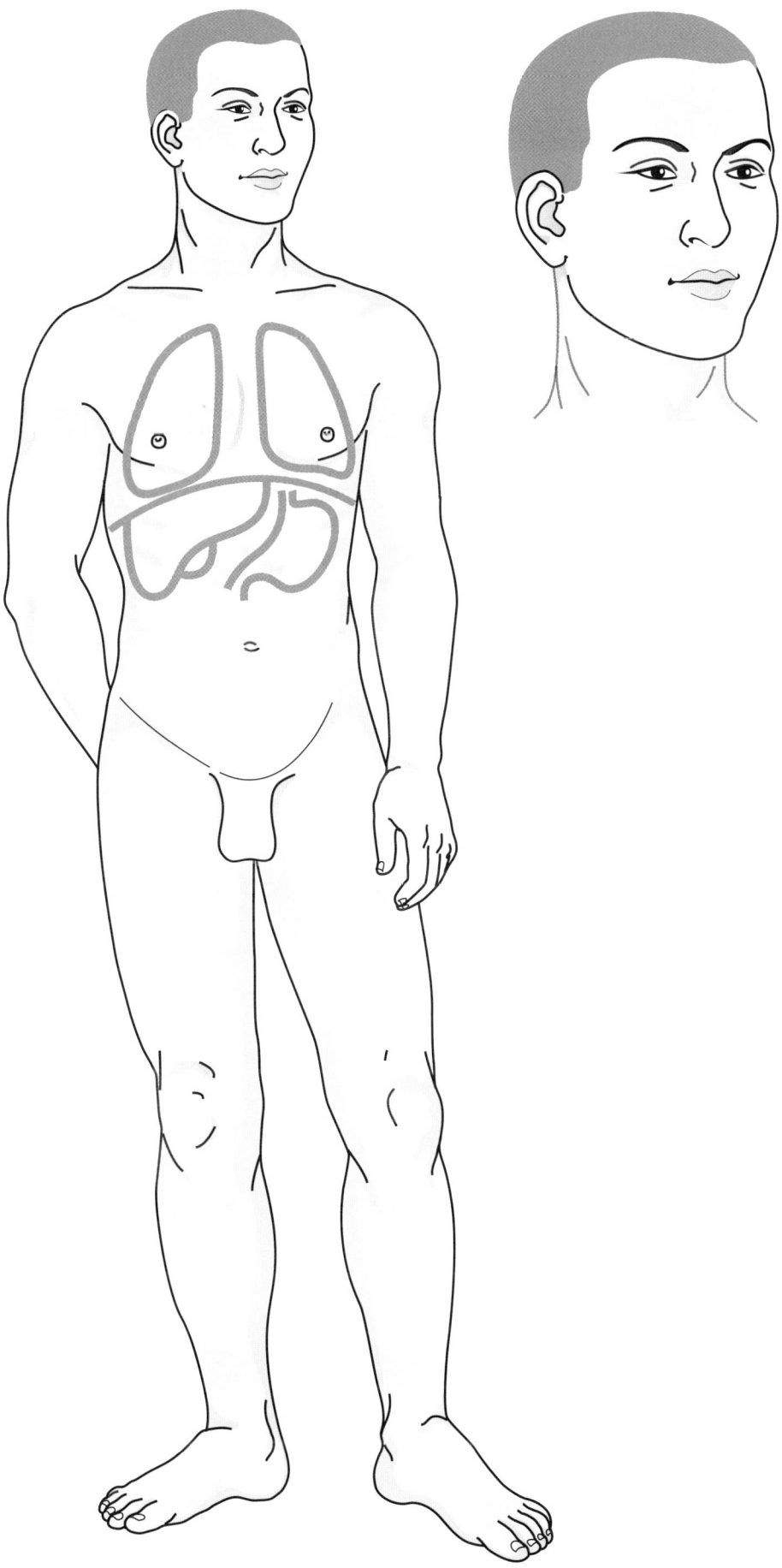

Figure 12.1 The Liver Channel — Stage 1

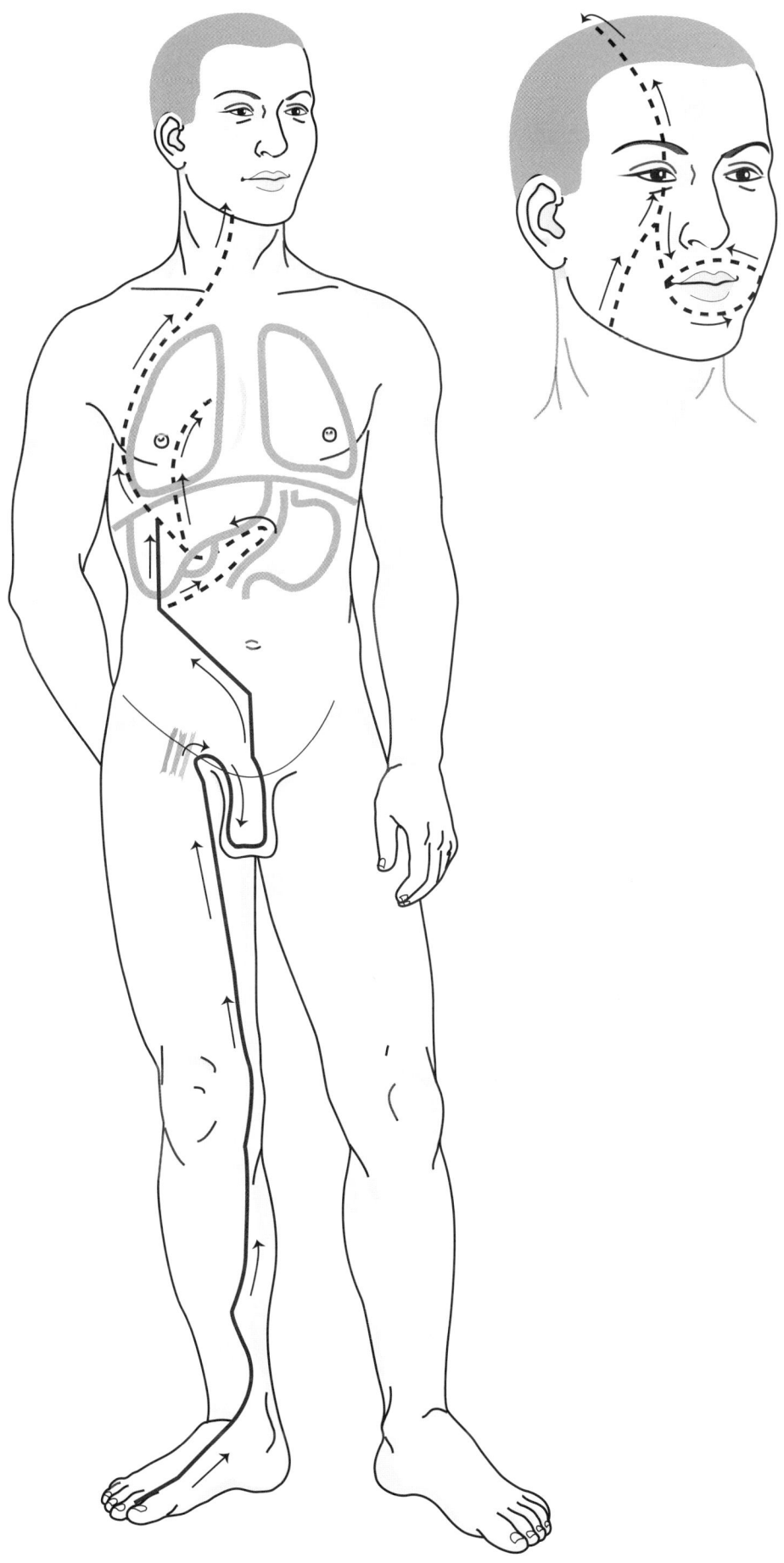

Figure 12.2 The Liver Channel — Stage 2

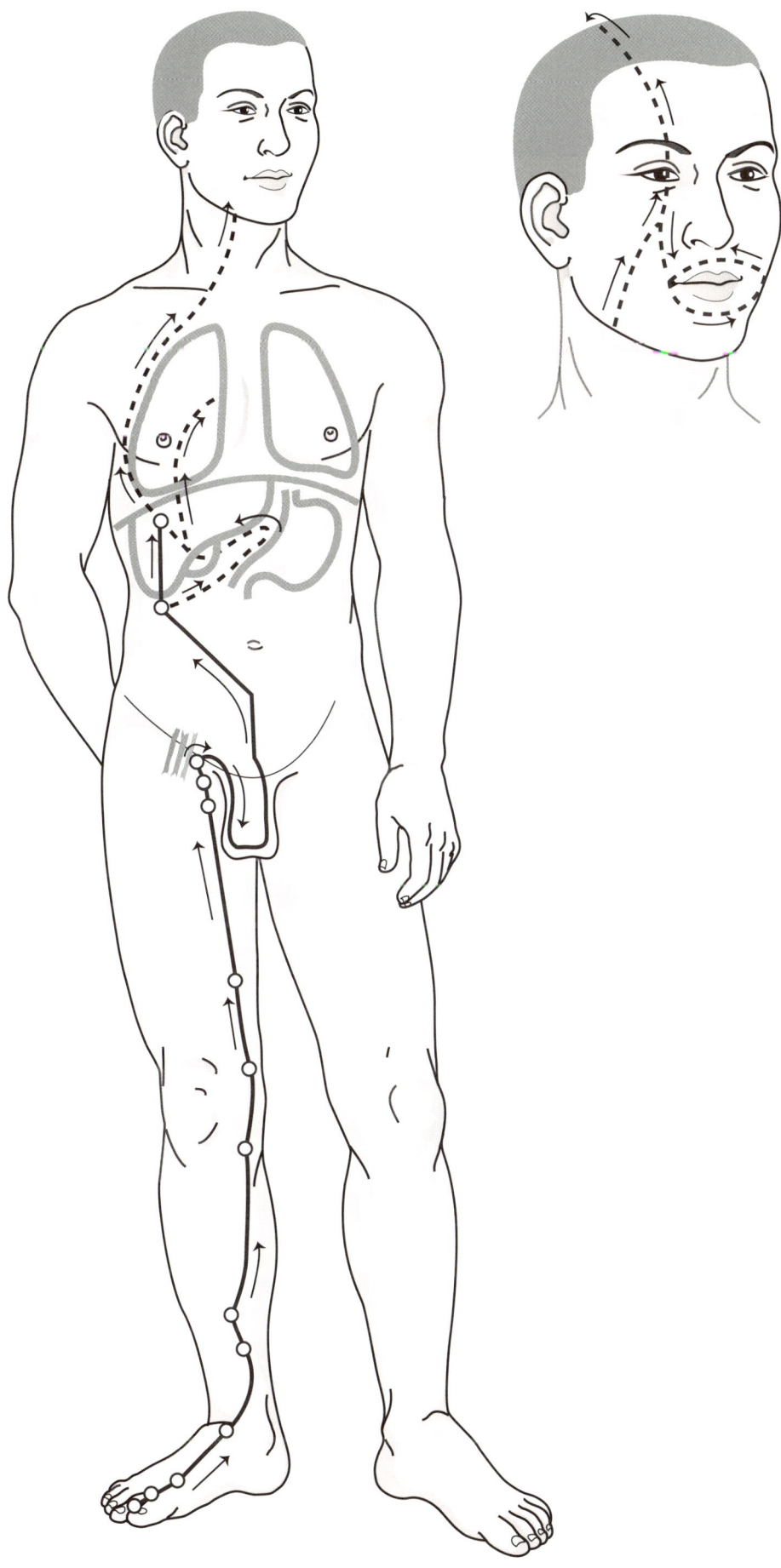

Figure 12.3 The Liver Channel — Stage 3

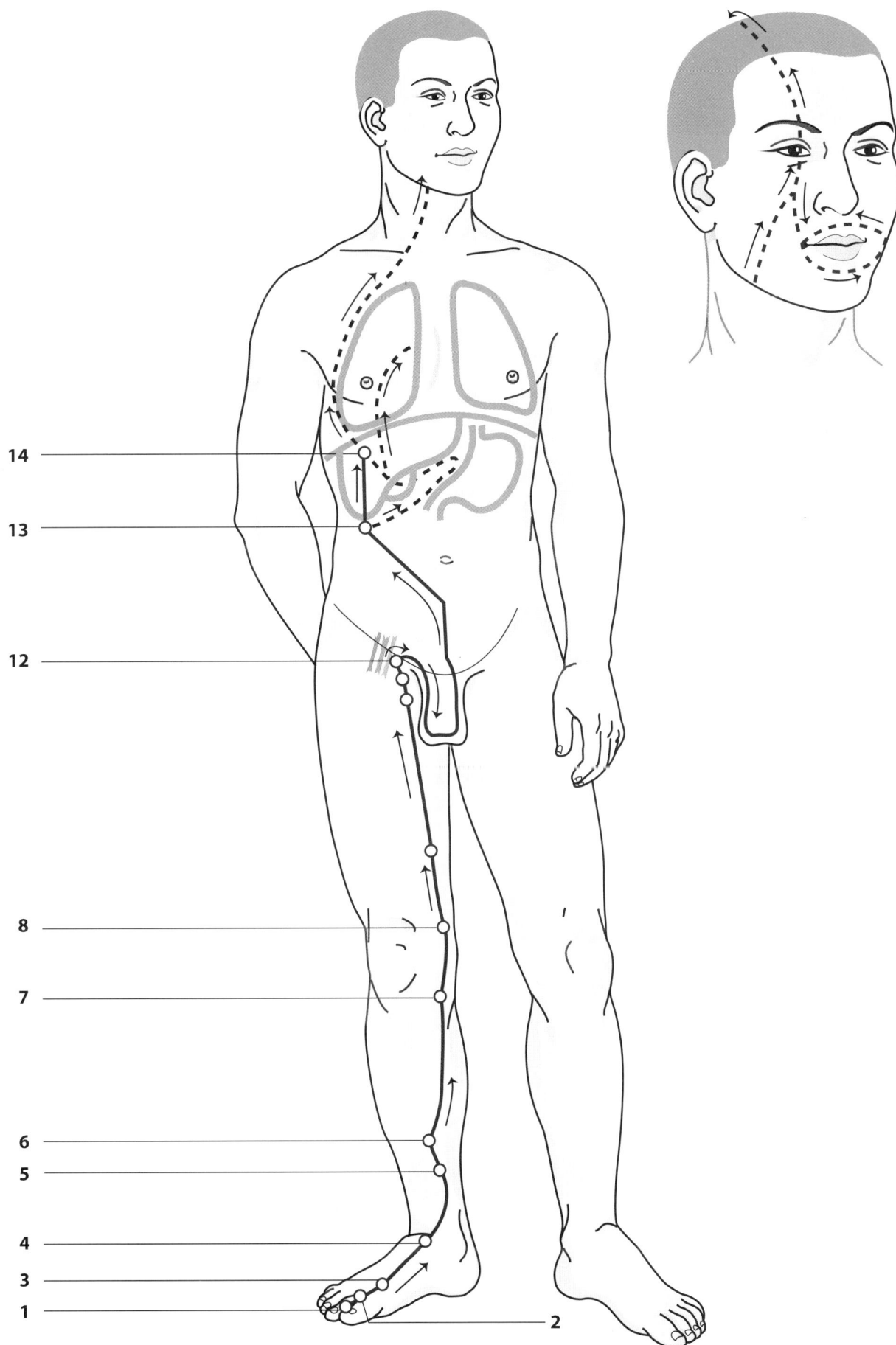

Figure 12.4 The Liver Channel — Stage 4

yuan — blue
luo — red
xi-cleft — green
five shu — yellow
lower he-sea — orange
back-shu — purple

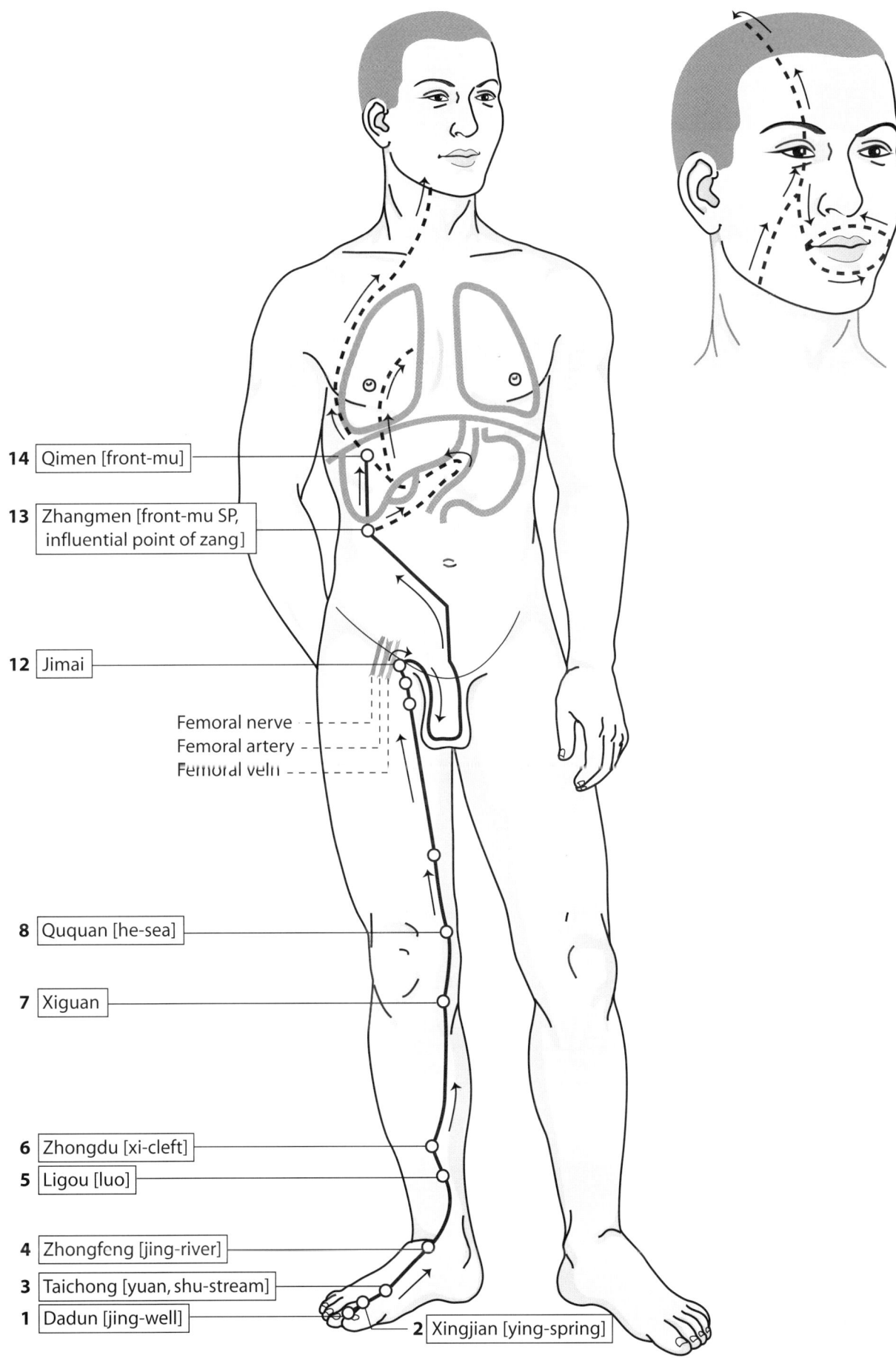

14 Qimen [front-mu]

13 Zhangmen [front-mu SP,
     influential point of zang]

12 Jimai

Femoral nerve
Femoral artery
Femoral vein

8 Ququan [he-sea]

7 Xiguan

6 Zhongdu [xi-cleft]
5 Ligou [luo]

4 Zhongfeng [jing-river]
3 Taichong [yuan, shu-stream]
1 Dadun [jing-well]

2 Xingjian [ying-spring]

Figure 12.5 The Liver Channel — Stage 5

THE LIVER CHANNEL — CASE STUDY

Ms VE, 25 year old planning a pregnancy

Ms VE has a regular 28-day cycle with 4 days of manageable bleeding. For about 10 days before menstruation she complains of mood swings, impatience, irritability, quick to anger, unhappiness, lumpy or swollen breasts, abdominal bloating and distension. With the onset of bleeding she experiences a 'dragging' feeling in her lower abdomen, cramping and referred back pain, which lasts 4–6 hours and is better for warmth. Her flow is dark red and sticky with medium-sized dark clots.

QUESTIONS

Circle or write your answers as required.

1   Is this an external or internal disorder?

2   If external:

(a) Is it due to heat or cold?

(b) Are there symptoms of wind, dampness or dryness?

(c) Is it acute, chronic or a mixed condition?

3   If internal:

(a) Is it due to deficiency or excess?

(i) If deficient, is it: qi, blood, jin ye, yin or yang?

(ii) If excess, is it: stagnant qi, stagnant blood, damp/phlegm, rebellious qi, rising liver yang, empty fire etc?

(b) Is it due to cold or heat?

(c) Which zang fu are affected?

(d) Which channels are affected?

4 **What might the pulse feel like?**
Describe: pulse rate, rhythm, depth, shape and strength.

5 **What might the tongue look like?**
Describe:
  – tongue body (colour, shape, thickness)
  – tongue coating (moisture, colour, thickness, distribution, root).

6 **What is the Chinese diagnosis?**
Where appropriate discuss the root (ben), the presenting symptoms (biao) and the five phase/wu xing dynamics (the relationship between and among the zang fu organs under syndromes of imbalance or disease).

7 **What is your treatment principle?**

8 **What points would you use and why? Include adjunctive therapy such as moxa or cupping if appropriate.**
(A minimum of five points, use only points on the Lung, Large Intestine, Stomach, Spleen, Heart, Small Intestine, Bladder, Kidney, Pericardium, San jiao, Gall Bladder and Liver Channels.)

Chapter Thirteen

THE EXTRAORDINARY VESSEL — REN MAI

奇经- 任脉

Ren Mai, together with Du Mai, are exceptional among the eight extraordinary vessels in that they have their own acupuncture points.

For this reason Ren Mai and Du Mai are often included with the 12 primary channels, and together are known as the '14 channels'.

Ren Mai and Du Mai are like *yin* and *yang* — Ren Mai goes to the front of the body (*yin*) and Du Mai to the back of the body (*yang*).

Ren Mai Vessel — conception

Li Shi Zhen, who described the most detailed trajectory for this vessel, believed that Ren Mai was the ocean or controller or confluence of the *yin* channels. According to the Spiritual Pivot, Ren Mai originates in the uterus in women (*bao gong*) and the Palace of Essence in men (*jing gong*).

Classically, points below the umbilicus are used to treat obstetrical and gynaecological disease; points between the umbilicus and Zhongwan Ren12 treat disorders of the San Jiao; and points above Zhongwan Ren12 treat disorders of the *shen*, respiratory patterns and the upper jiao.

The Ren Mai Channel allows direct access to the *zang fu*. Six of the front-*mu* points are located on this channel and allow direct access to the bladder (Zhongji Ren3), small intestine (Guanyuan Ren4), san jiao (Shimen Ren5), stomach (Zhongwan Ren12), heart (Juque Ren14) and pericardium (Shanzhong Ren17). These important points regulate their *zang fu*.

The main pathway:

- originates from the uterus in females and lower abdomen in males and emerges in the perineum at Huiyin Ren1
- travels anteriorly to the pubic region, goes upwards along the midline of the abdomen and continues to ascend up the chest, throat and jaw
- enters the body at the mento-labial groove at Chengjiang Ren24.

The other branches:

- a branch arises in the pelvic cavity, descends and enters the spine, then travels upward inside the spinal column and ends in the lower jaw

- at Chengjiang Ren24, a branch encircles the mouth, with two smaller branches travelling up from each corner of the mouth through the cheek to enter the infraorbital region, ending below the eye at Chengqi ST1.

The coalescent points for Ren mai are:

Chengqi ST1, Yinjiao Du28

REN MAI CHANNEL POINTS			
WHO number	Pinyin	Name	Specific functions
Ren1	**Huiyin**	Meeting of Yin	
Ren2	**Qugu**	Curved Bone	
Ren3	**Zhongji**	Central Pole	Front-Mu (BL)
Ren4	**Guanyuan**	Origin Pass	Front-Mu (SI)
Ren5	**Shimen**	Stone Gate	Front-Mu (SJ)
Ren6	**Qihai**	Sea of Qi	
Ren7	**Yinjiao**	Yin Intersection	
Ren8	**Shenque**	Spirit Gate	
Ren9	**Shuifen**	Water Divide	
Ren10	**Xiawan**	Lower Vent	
Ren11	Jianli	Interior Strengthening	
Ren12	**Zhongwan**	Central Vent	Front-Mu (ST), Influential Point of Fu
Ren13	Shangwan	Upper Vent	
Ren14	**Juque**	Great Tower Gate	Front-Mu (HT)
Ren15	**Jiuwei**	Turtle Dove Tail	Luo-Connecting
Ren16	Zhongting	Centre Palace	
Ren17	**Shanzhong**	Chest Centre	Front-Mu (PC), Influential Point of Qi
Ren18	Yutang	Jade Hall	
Ren19	Zigong	Purple Palace	
Ren20	Huagai	Florid Canopy	
Ren21	Xuanji	Jade Pivot	
Ren22	**Tiantu**	Celestial Chimney	
Ren23	**Lianquan**	Ridge Spring	
Ren24	**Chengjiang**	Source Receptacle	

Note: The 17 points highlighted in bold are provided on the composite diagram for this channel (the fifth diagram).

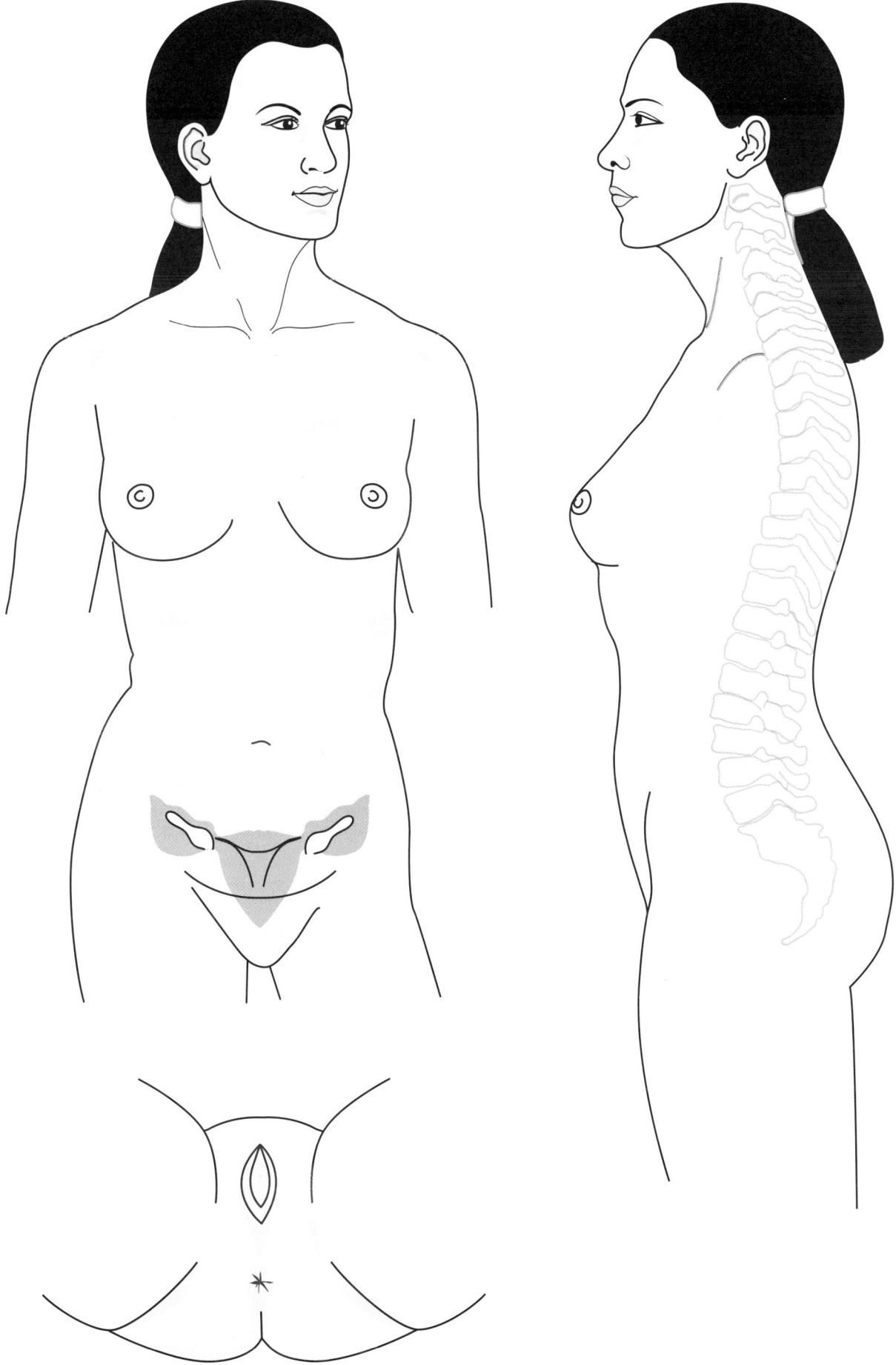

Figure 13.1 Ren Vessel — Stage 1

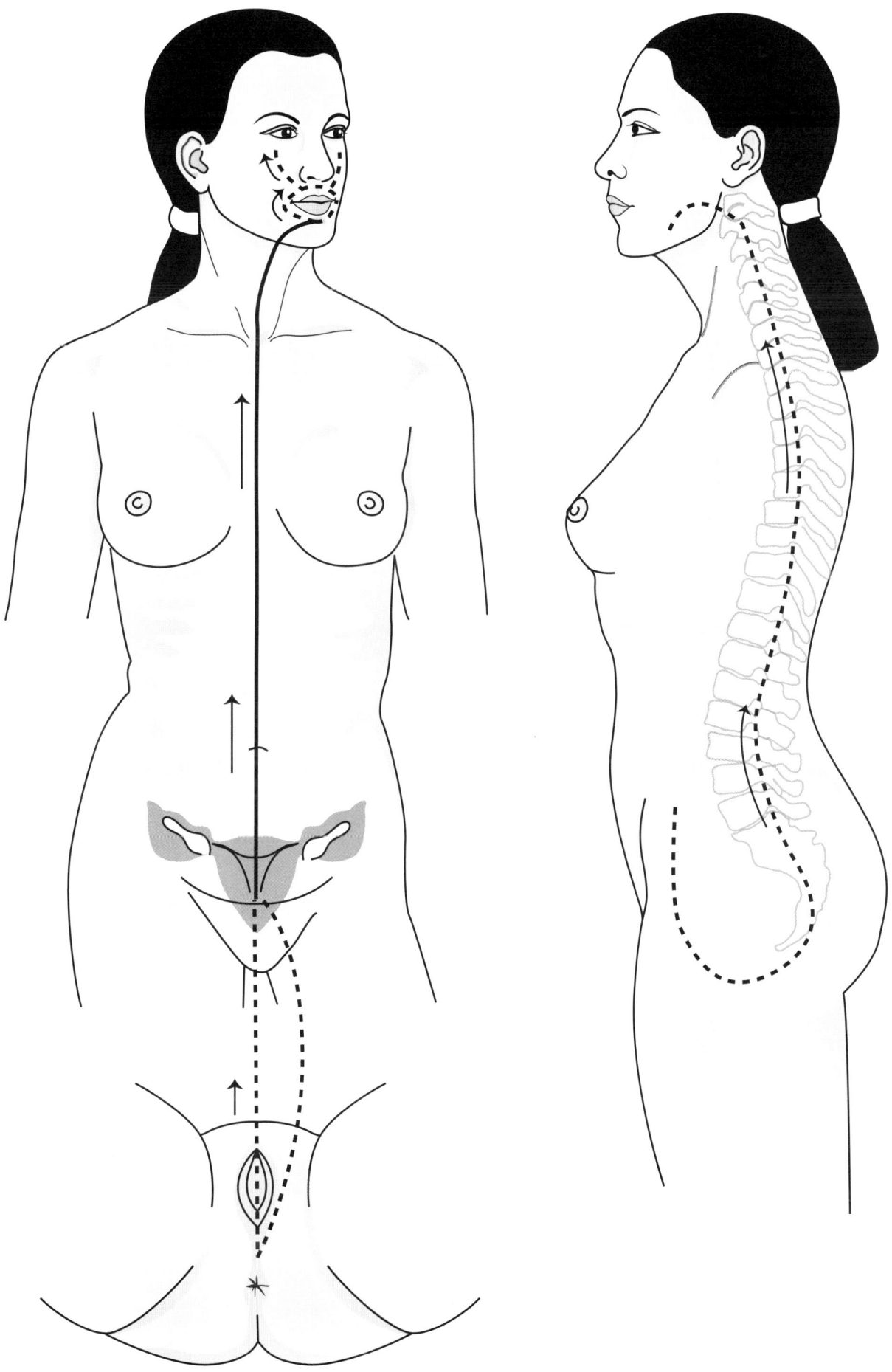

Figure 13.2 Ren Vessel — Stage 2

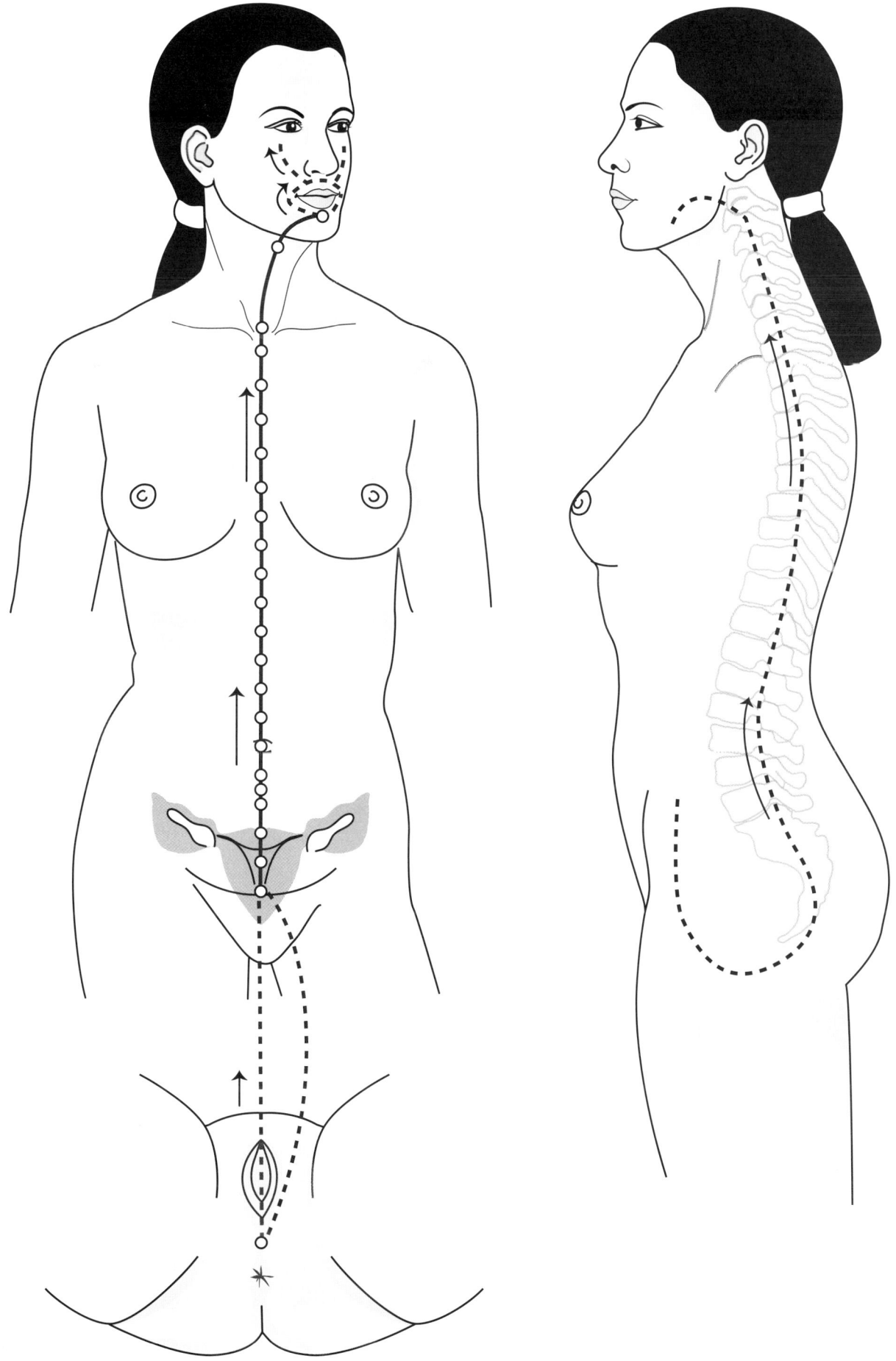

Figure 13.3 Ren Vessel — Stage 3

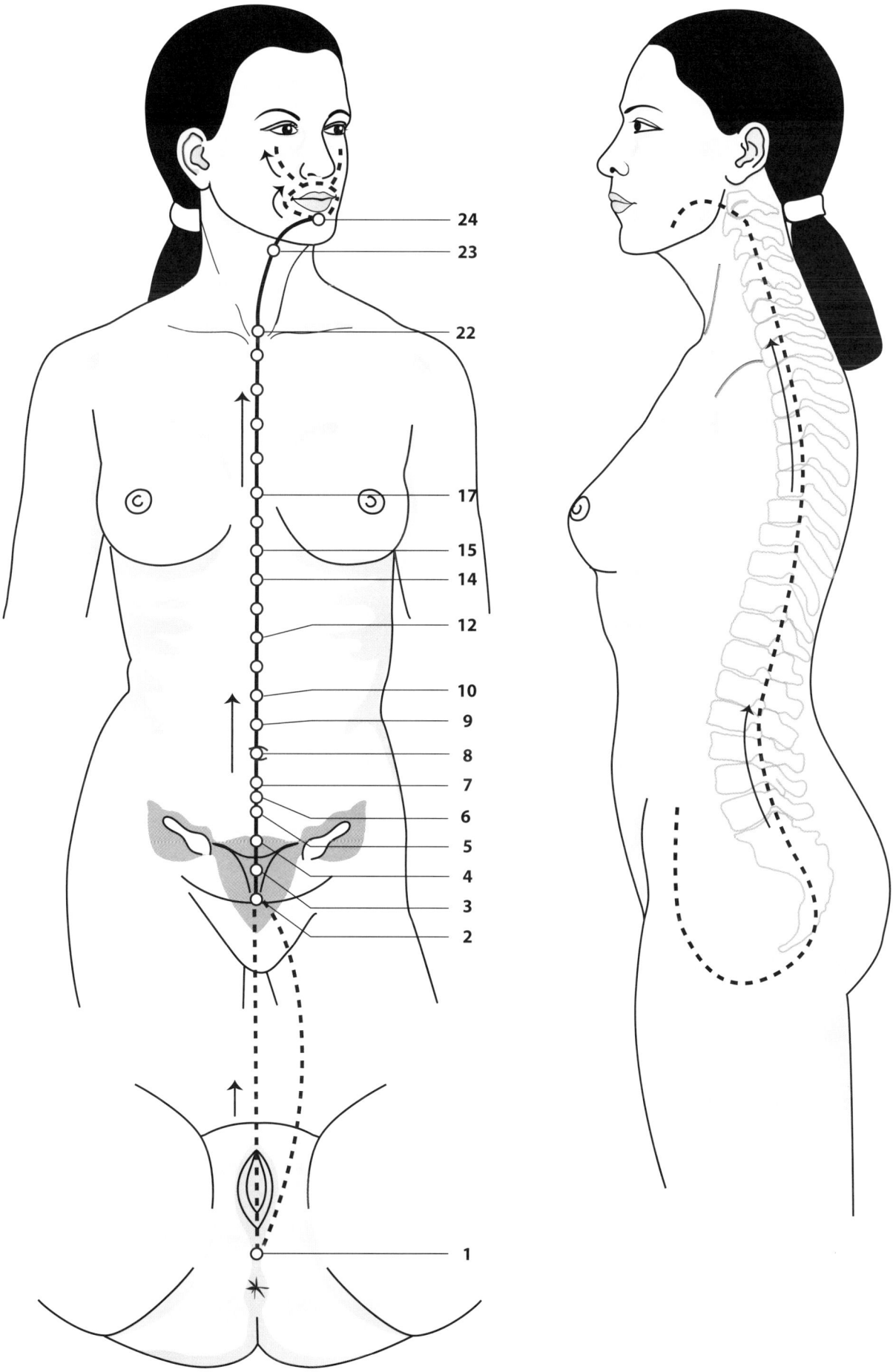

Figure 13.4 Ren Vessel — Stage 4

yuan — blue	
luo — red	
xi-cleft — green	
five shu — yellow	
lower he-sea — orange	
back-shu — purple	

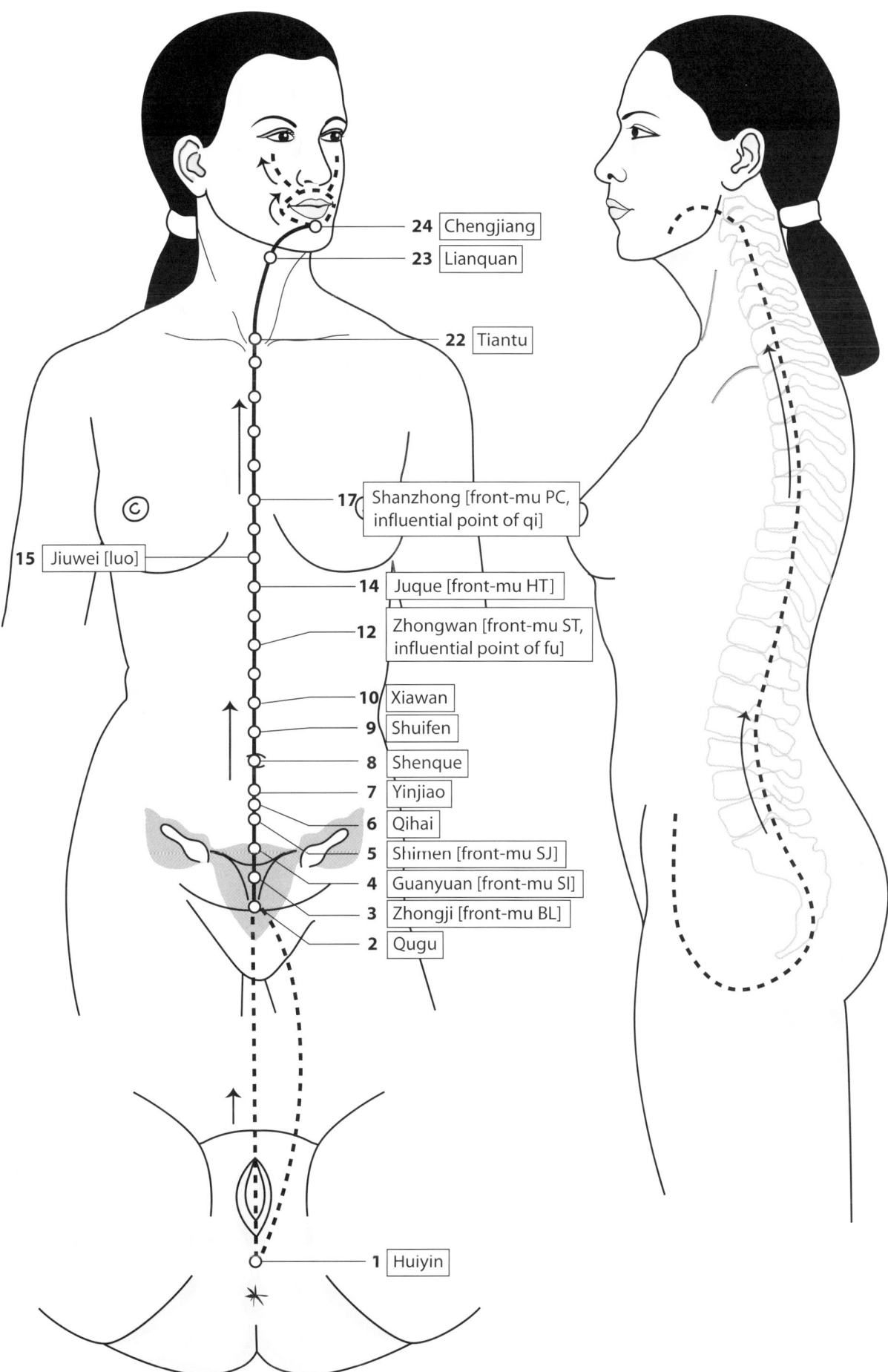

24 Chengjiang
23 Lianquan
22 Tiantu
17 Shanzhong [front-mu PC, influential point of qi]
15 Jiuwei [luo]
14 Juque [front-mu HT]
12 Zhongwan [front-mu ST, influential point of fu]
10 Xiawan
9 Shuifen
8 Shenque
7 Yinjiao
6 Qihai
5 Shimen [front-mu SJ]
4 Guanyuan [front-mu SI]
3 Zhongji [front-mu BL]
2 Qugu
1 Huiyin

Figure 13.5 Ren Vessel Channel — Stage 5

Clinical use of extraordinary channels

1. Use of individual channels

Ren mai and Du Mai Channels have their own points, which can be used specifically for a particular problem.

Each of the eight extraordinary channels can be used individually, by using the confluent or master point, to treat failure of any of their functions. For example, Zulingqi GB41, the master point for Dai Mai, can be used for vaginitis due to liver or gall bladder *damp heat* (see diagram on next page showing functions of the extraordinary channel pairs).

2. Use of extraordinary channel pairs

The principles are simplicity and harmony.

(a) Use only the master points of a pair. This will treat complex conditions involving two or more organs with minimum needles to obtain powerful results. Each pair can treat a group of channels or a group of organs and is associated with a particular constitutional and personality type.

(b) A powerful combination can be achieved by combining master points with points on Du Mai or Ren Mai Channels. For example, for a client with cold hands and feet due to deficient kidney qi and dantian energy, Gongsun SP4 and Neiguan PC6 can be combined with reinforcing method and moxa on Guanyuan Ren4.

(c) There are various methods of using master points. Personal preference and an intuitive assessment of the needs of a particular client may determine the method used. Master points of both channels of the pair can be used bilaterally or unilaterally.

Needles are removed in reverse order to insertion.

Bilateral use — needles are inserted on both sides for each master point and additional points can be used bilaterally.

Unilateral use — when treating a man, the master point of the primary channel is needed first, on the left side, followed by the master point of the secondary channel on the right side. The reverse applies for a female (right side, then left side).

Unilateral use of the affected side — if a problem is solely or predominantly on one side of the body then the master points of both channels can be used on the affected side only. For example, a right-sided liver headache and right-sided hypochondriac pain can be treated with Zulingqi GB41 and Waiguan SJ5 on the right side only. This treatment must be modified if kidney or liver yin xu is present. Balance the treatment with an additional point such as Saninjiao SP6 or Taixi KI3.

Functions of the extraordinary channel pairs

Channels used include both the main channels on the external pathway of the extraordinary channel and the channels of the confluent/master points.

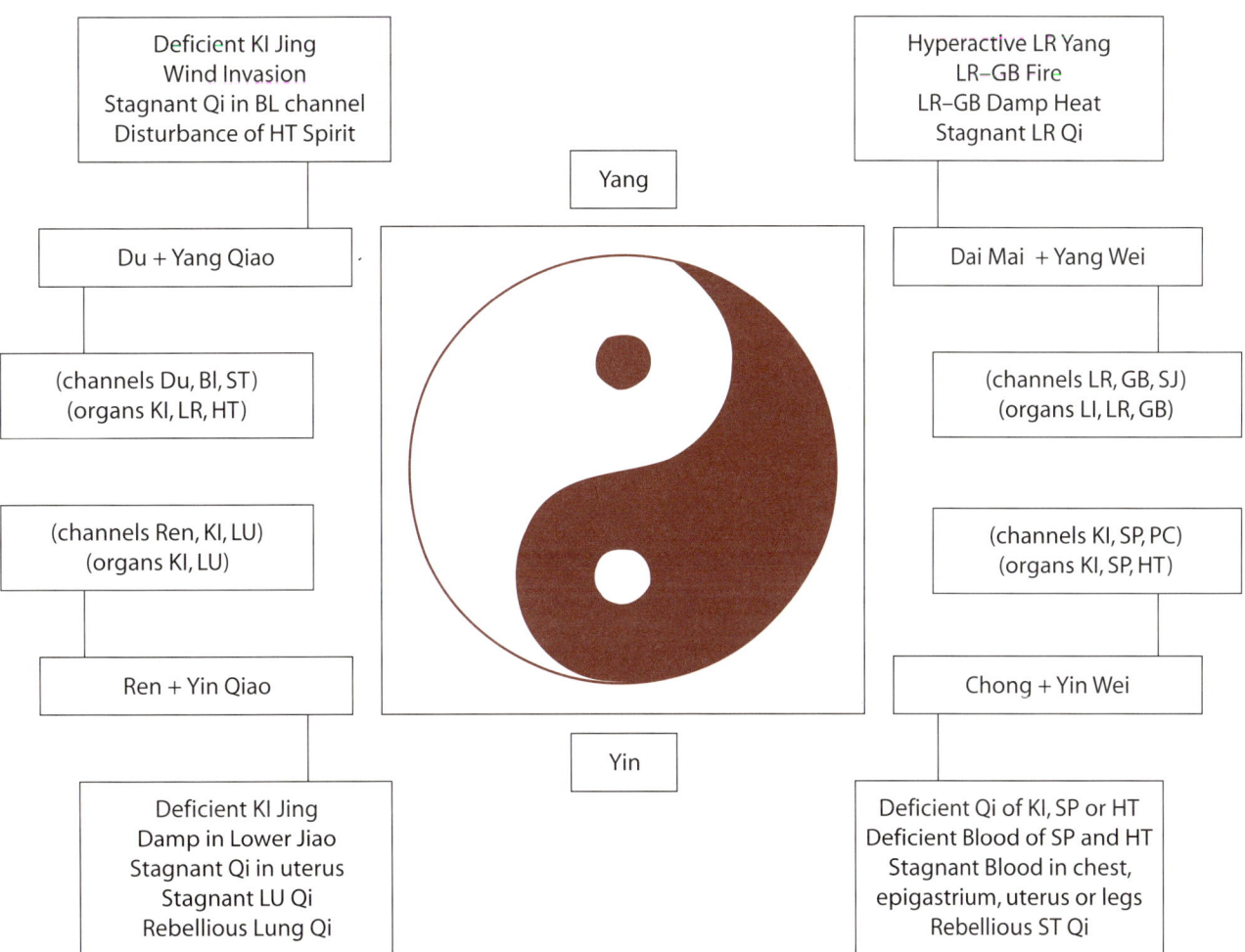

Modified from Ross J, 1995. Acupuncture Point Combinations: The Key to Clinical Success. Churchill Livingstone, London, UK. P. 106.

REN MAI — CASE STUDY

Ms LB, 28 year old business executive

Ms LB is considering a hysterectomy (removal of the womb) to control four years of severe pain from endometriosis. Two years ago she had surgery to remove extensive endometriosis from many sites in her pelvic cavity and a chocolate cyst from one ovary. She was pain-free for 6 months after surgery. Now, she describes her periods as 'heavy and painful', but it is the knife-like stabbing pain (10/10) in her abdomen and anus at mid-cycle lasting for 4–5 days that she can no longer tolerate. Her cycle is 26 days, with a heavy, fresh red flow, medium clots, a stabbing pain (6/10) radiating into the pelvis and top of thighs on the first day of bleeding, tiredness, and generally feeling cold. For up to a week prior to menstruation she has increasing clear vaginal secretions (leucorrhoea).

QUESTIONS

Circle or write your answers as required.

1   Is this an external or internal disorder?

2   If external:

(a) Is it due to heat or cold?

(b) Are there symptoms of wind, dampness or dryness?

(c) Is it acute, chronic or a mixed condition?

3   If internal:

(a) Is it due to deficiency or excess?

    (i)   If deficient, is it: qi, blood, jin ye, yin or yang?

    (ii) If excess, is it: stagnant ai, stagnant blood, damp/phlegm, rebellious qi, rising liver yang, empty fire etc?

(b) Is it due to cold or heat?

(c) Which zang fu are affected?

(d) Which channels are affected?

4 What might the pulse feel like?

Describe: pulse rate, rhythm, depth, shape and strength.

5 What might the tongue look like?

Describe:

– tongue body (colour, shape, thickness)

– tongue coating (moisture, colour, thickness, distribution, root).

6 What is the Chinese diagnosis?

Where appropriate discuss the root (ben), the presenting symptoms (biao) and the five phase/ wu xing dynamics (the relationship between and among the zang fu organs under syndromes of imbalance or disease).

7 What is your treatment principle?

8 What points would you use and why? Include any adjunctive therapy such as moxa or cupping, if appropriate.

(A minimum of five points, use points on any of the primary channels and Ren Mai.)

Chapter Fourteen

THE EXTRAORDINARY VESSEL —
DU MAI

奇经-督脉

Du Mai is the 'sea of the *yang* channels'.

As Du mai ascends along the spine, its points have the ability to treat diseases of the *zang fu*, roughly corresponding to their location. Many of its points treat exterior or wind disorders, disorders of the sense organs, disorders of the heart, and disorders of the brain and spirit. Du Mai is the channel that mediates between the brain and the heart.

The main pathway:

*   originates in the lower abdomen and emerges from the perineum at Changqiang Du1

*   travels posteriorly along the midline of the sacrum and ascends internally alongside the spinal column to Fengfu Du16 at the nape of the neck where it enters the brain (see other branches)

*   continues over the head through Baihui Du20 and then descends down the midline of the head, forehead and nose to the philtrum at Renzhong Du26, ending at the junction of the upper lip and gum.

The other branches:

*   a branch enters the brain at Fengfu Du16 and ascends to Baihui Du20 at the vertex

*   another branch originates in the lower abdomen, descends to the genitals and perineum, encircles the anus and ascends inside the spinal column to enter the kidneys

*   a second branch originates in the lower abdomen, encircles the external genitalia, ascends to the middle of the umbilicus, runs upward over the chest passing through the heart, continues up through the throat, encircles the mouth and ascends to below the middle of the eyes

- two other branches arise at Jingming BL1 above the inner canthus of the eye and follow the Bladder Channel bilaterally along the forehead, converge at the vertex at Baihui Du20 to enter the brain, and re-emerge as a single channel at Fengfu Du16, then divide again, each descending through Fengmen BL12 and running along either side of the spine to end in the kidneys.

The coalescent points of Du Mai are:

Fengmen BL12, Huiyin Ren1

DU MAI CHANNEL POINTS

WHO number	Pinyin	Name	Specific functions
Du1	**Changqiang**	Long Strong	Luo-Connecting
Du2	**Yaoshu**	Lumbar Shu	
Du3	**Yaoyangguan**	Lumbar Yang Pass	
Du4	**Mingmen**	Life Gate	
Du5	Xuanshu	Suspended Pivot	
Du6	Jizhong	Spinal Centre	
Du7	Zhongshu	Central Pivot	
Du8	Jinsuo	Sinew Contraction	
Du9	**Zhiyang**	Extremity of Yang	
Du10	**Lingtai**	Spirit Tower	
Du11	**Shendao**	Spirit Path	
Du12	**Shenzhu**	Body Pillar	
Du13	**Taodao**	Kiln Path	
Du14	**Dazhui**	Great Hammer	
Du15	**Yamen**	Mute's Gate	
Du16	**Fengfu**	Wind Mansion	
Du17	Naohu	Brain's Door	
Du18	Qiangjian	Unyielding Space	
Du19	Houding	Behind the Vertex	
Du20	**Baihui**	Hundred Convergences	
Du21	Qianding	Before the Vertex	
Du22	Xinhui	Fontanelle Meeting	
Du23	**Shangxing**	Upper Star	
Du24	**Shenting**	Spirit Court	
Du25	Suliao	White Bone-Hole	
Du26	**Renzhong**	Water Trough	
Du27	Duiduan	Extremity of the Mouth	
Du28	Yinjiao	Gum Intersection	

Note: The 16 points highlighted in bold are provided on the composite diagram for this channel (the fifth diagram).

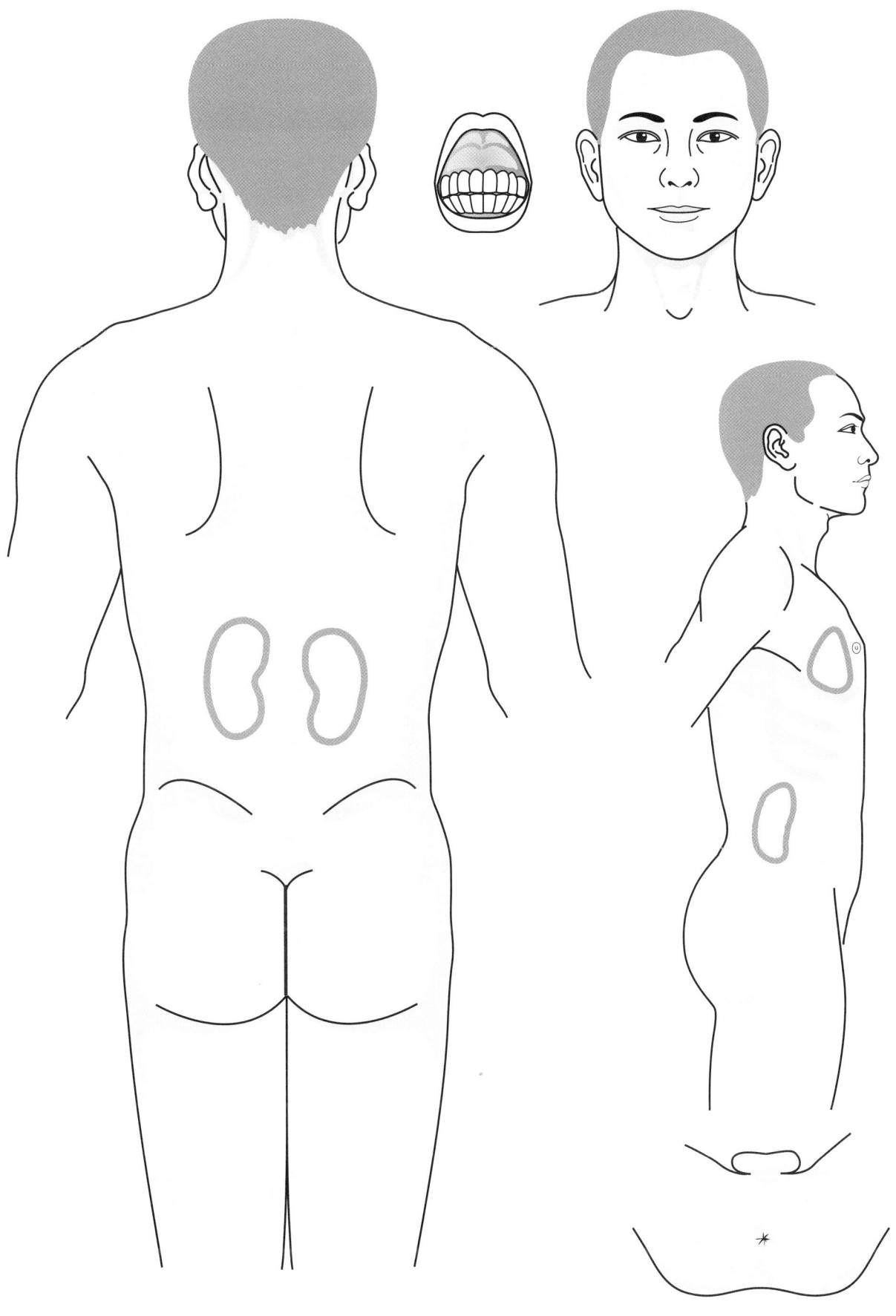

Figure 14.1 Du Mai Channel — Stage 1

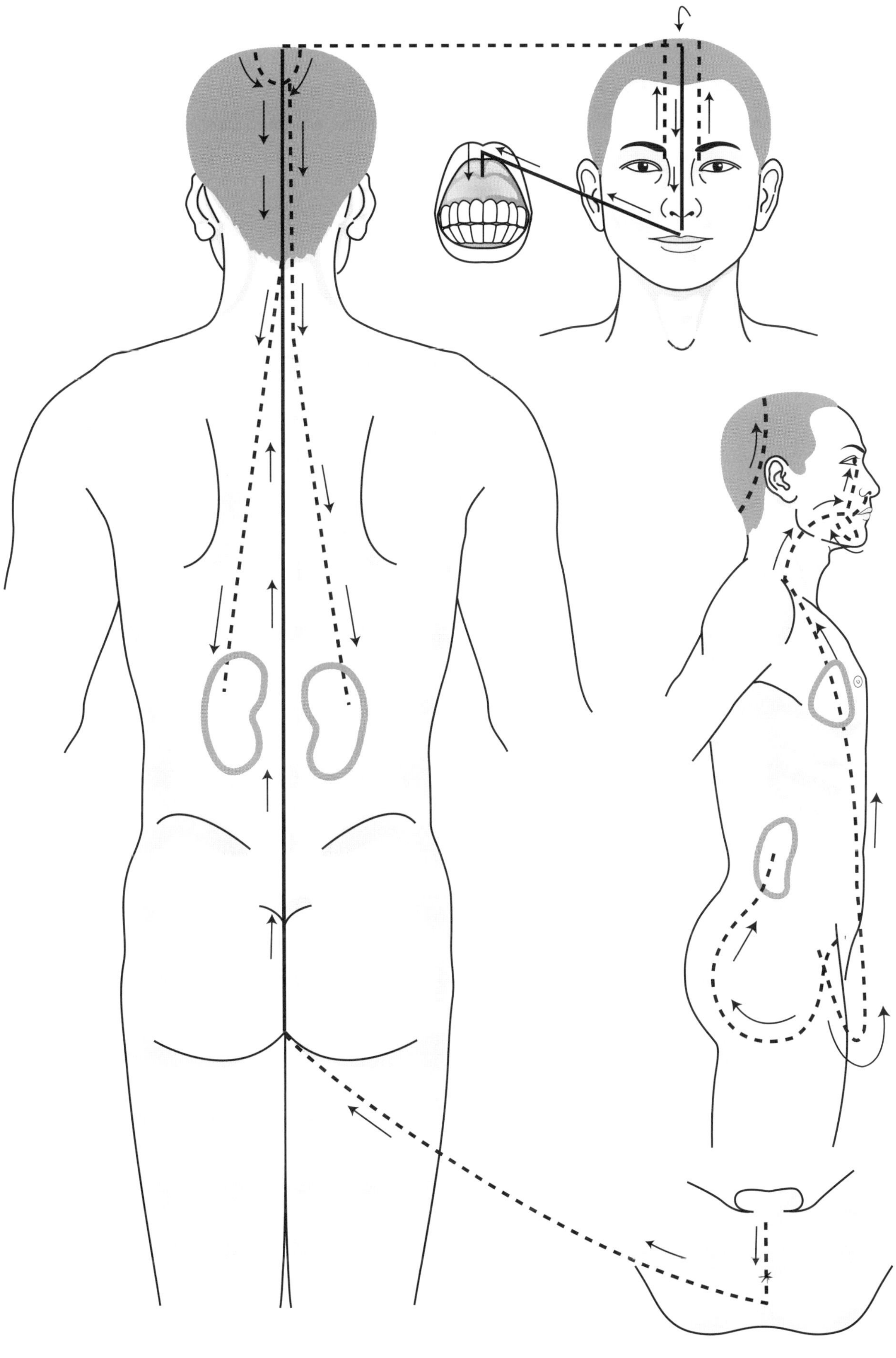

Figure 14.2 Du Mai Channel — Stage 2

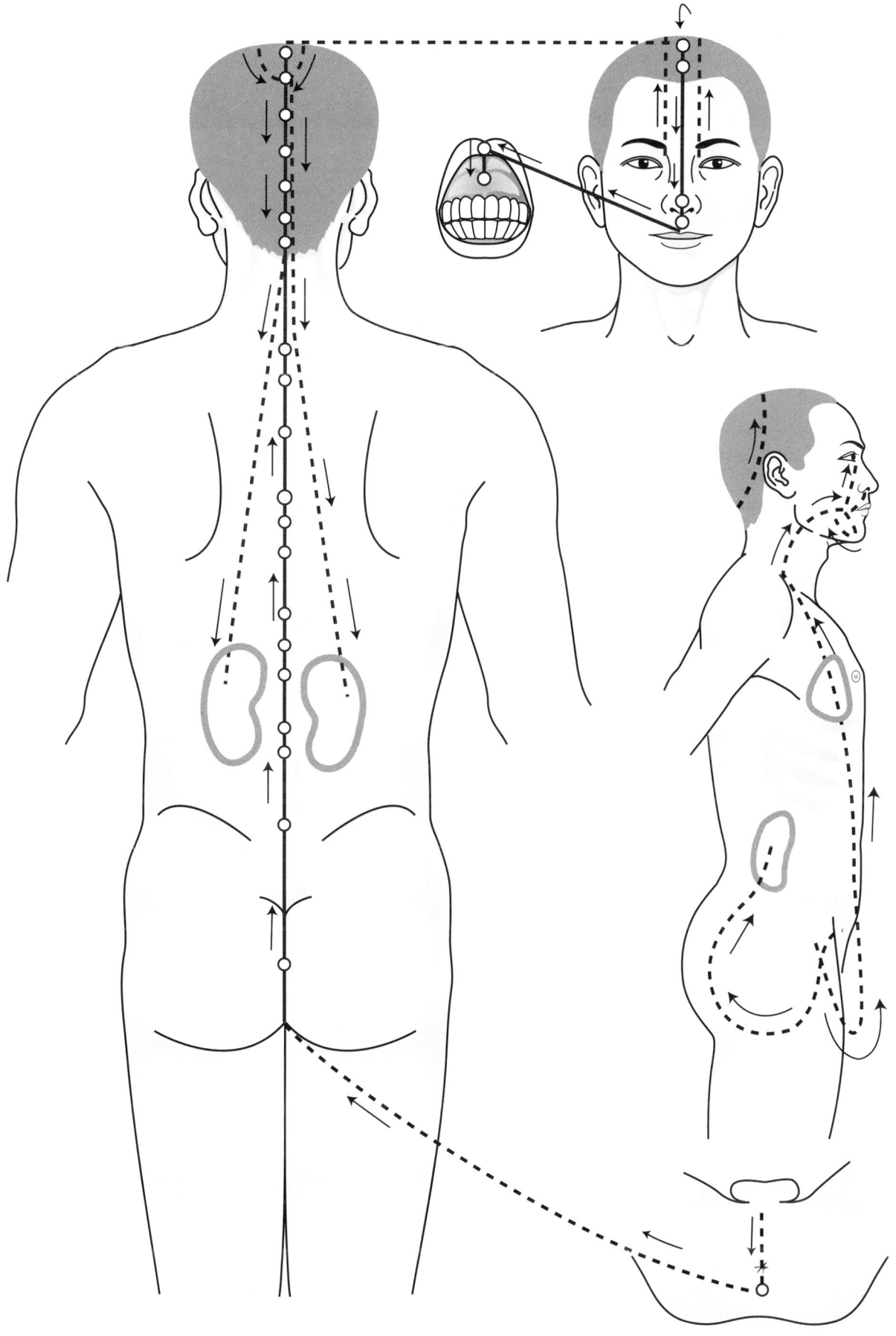

Figure 14.3 Du Mai Channel — Stage 3

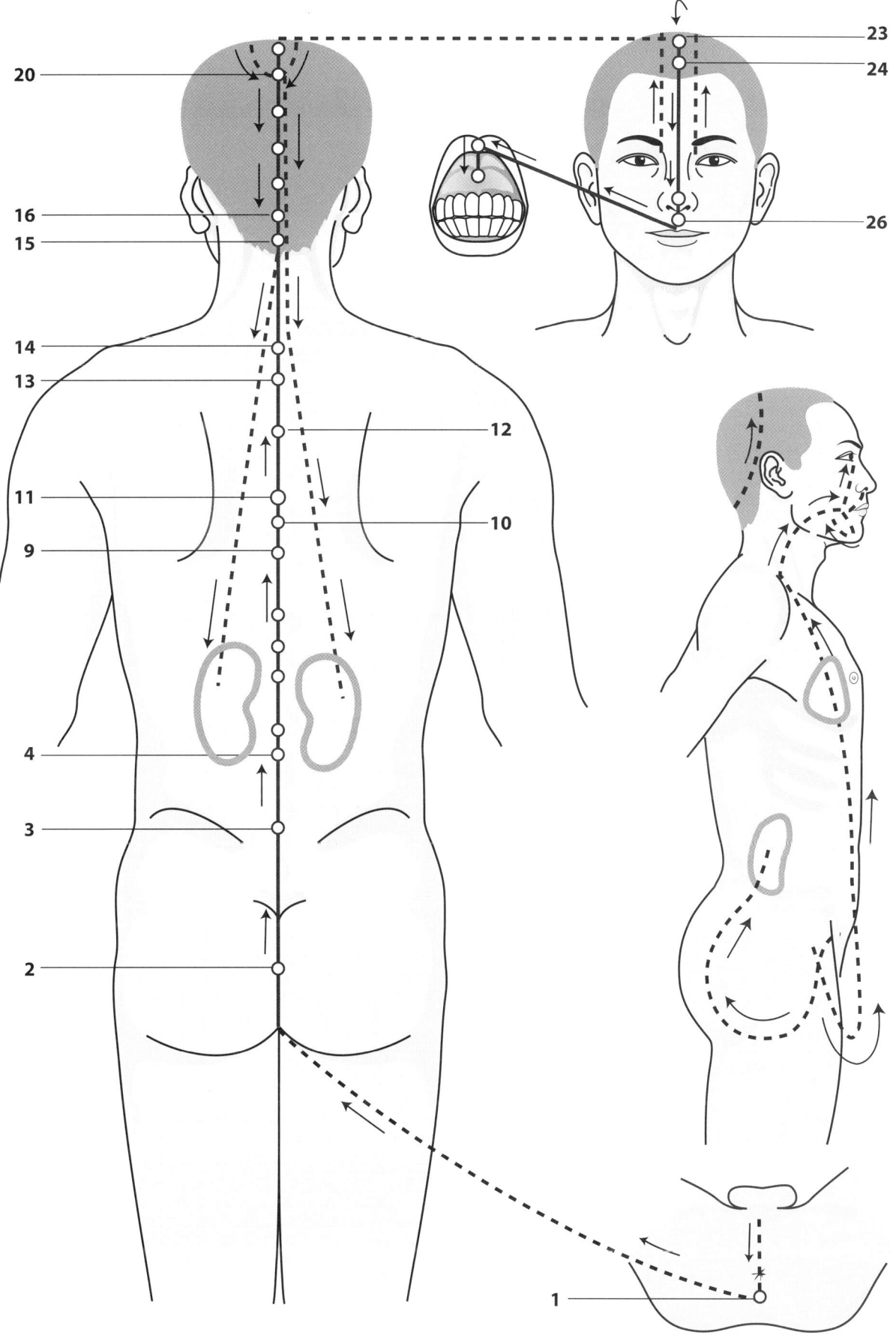

Figure 14.4 Du Mai Channel — Stage 4

yuan — blue	
luo — red	
xi-cleft — green	
five shu — yellow	
lower he-sea — orange	
back-shu — purple	

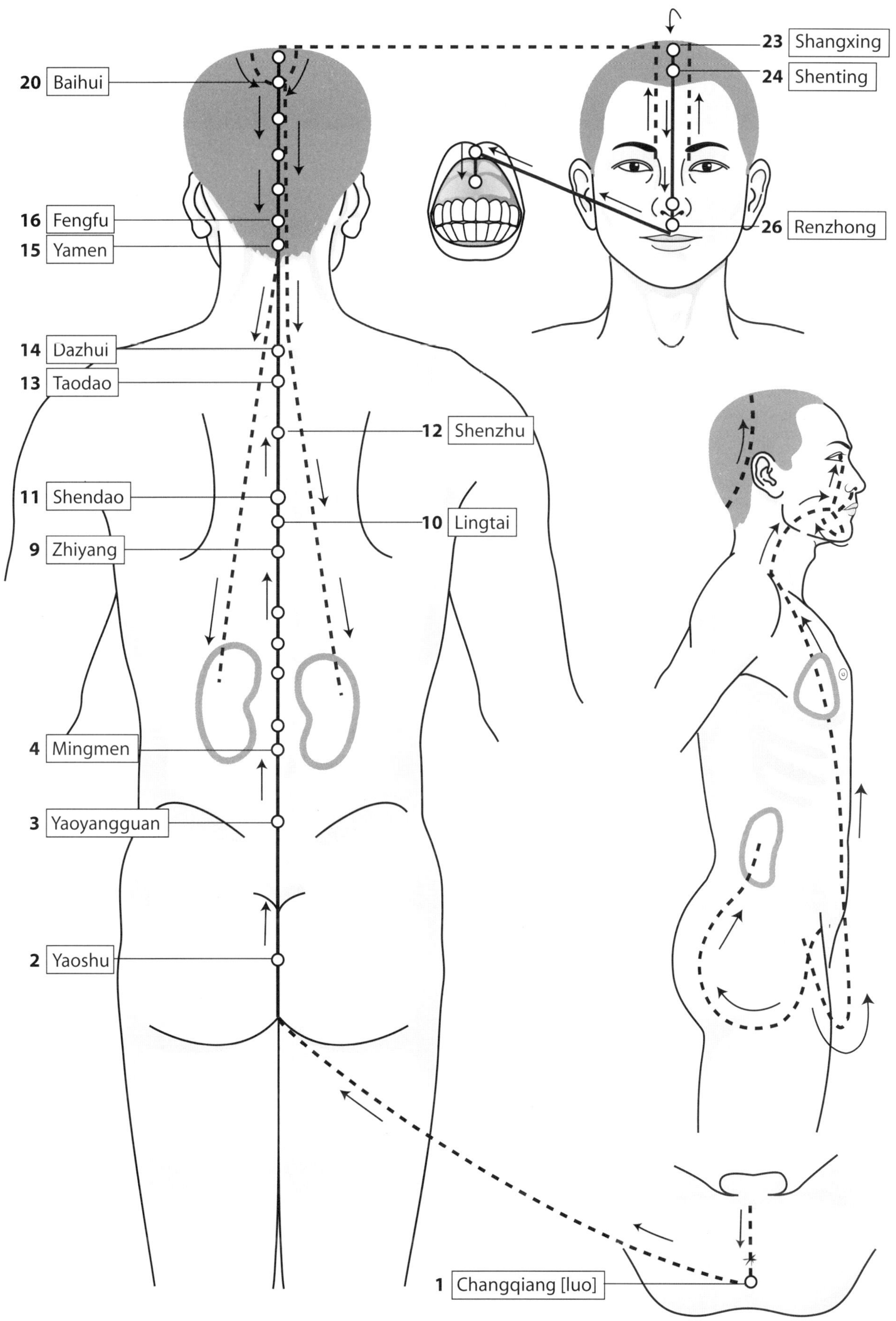

23 Shangxing

24 Shenting

20 Baihui

26 Renzhong

16 Fengfu

15 Yamen

14 Dazhui

13 Taodao

12 Shenzhu

11 Shendao

10 Lingtai

9 Zhiyang

4 Mingmen

3 Yaoyangguan

2 Yaoshu

1 Changqiang [luo]

Figure 14.5 Du Mai Channel — Stage 5

DU MAI — CASE STUDY

Mr AF, 36 year old landscape gardener

Mr AF presents with a 3-year history of chronic back ache that he rates 4–5/10, and which is centred over the spine in the lumbar area. He complains of chronic stiffness, worse in the morning, achy back pain aggravated by work and better for rest and heat. Other symptoms include loss of appetite, tiredness, feeling apathetic, loose stools, nocturia (1–2x night), aversion to cold, cold limbs, weak cold knees, and reduced libido.

QUESTIONS

Circle or write your answers as required.

1   Is this an external or internal disorder?

2   If external:
   (a) Is it due to heat or cold?

   (b) Are there symptoms of wind, dampness or dryness?

   (c) Is it acute, chronic or a mixed condition?

3   If internal:
   (a) Is it due to deficiency or excess?

      (i)   If deficient, is it: qi, blood, jin ye, yin or yang?

      (ii) If excess, is it: stagnant qi, stagnant blood, damp/phlegm, rebellious qi, rising liver yang, empty fire etc?

   (b) Is it due to cold or heat?

   (c) Which zang fu are affected?

   (d) Which channels are affected?

4 What might the pulse feel like?
   Describe: pulse rate, rhythm, depth, shape and strength.

5 What might the tongue look like?
   Describe:
   – tongue body (colour, shape, thickness)
   – tongue coating (moisture, colour, thickness, distribution, root).

6 What is the Chinese diagnosis?
   Where appropriate discuss the root (ben), the presenting symptoms (biao) and the five phase/ wu xing dynamics (the relationship between and among the zang fu organs under syndromes of imbalance or disease).

7 What is your treatment principle?

8 What points would you use and why? Include any adjunctive therapy such as moxa or cupping, if appropriate.
   (A minimum of five points, use points on any of the 12 primary channels, Ren Mai and Du Mai.)

Chapter Fifteen

THE OTHER SIX EXTRAORDINARY VESSELS AND EXTRA POINTS

其它：六奇经和奇穴

While Ren Mai and Du Mai have their own acupuncture points, the other six extraordinary vessels have no points of their own, passing instead through the points on the 14 channels. These points are referred to as the 'coalescent points'.

Chong Mai — penetrating

Chong mai is known as the 'Sea of Blood' or the 'Sea of the 12 primary channels'.

It links the Stomach and Kidney Channels as well as strengthening the link between Ren Mai and Du Mai.

The main pathway:

- emerges through Qichong ST30 and communicates medially with the Kidney Channel at Henggu KI11 (see other branches)
- runs up both sides of the abdomen through the Kidney Channel points to Youmen KI21
- disperses into each side of the chest (see other branches).

The other branches:

- one branch originates in the uterus in women and inside the lower abdomen in men, and emerges in the perineum at Huiyin Ren1

- a branch ascends from Huiyin Ren1, enters the spine and travels upward inside the spinal column

- another branch ascends up each side of the chest, runs up along the sides of the throat, encircles the mouth, continues up alongside the nose and ends below the eye in the infraorbital region

- the leg branch emerges at Qichong ST30, descends along the medial aspect of the leg to the popliteal fossa, continues down the medial side of the lower leg, runs posterior to the medial malleolus and ends at the arch on the sole of the foot

- another branch separates from the leg branch posterior to the medial malleolus, and continues along the antero-medial aspect of the foot to end at the big toe.

The coalescent points are:

Huiyin Ren1, Yinjiao Ren7, Qichong ST30, Henggu KI11, Dahe KI12, Qixue KI13, Siman KI14, Zhongzhu KI15, Huangshu KI16, Shangqu KI17, Shiguan KI18, Yindu KI19, Futonggu KI20, Youmen KI21

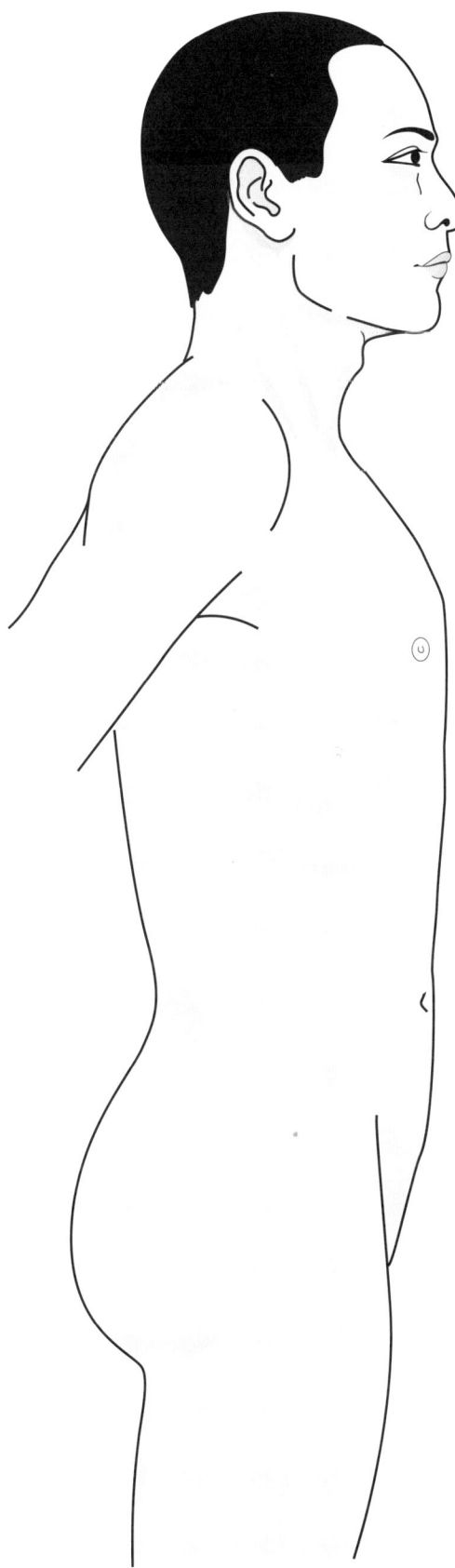

Figure 15.1 Chong Mai Channel — Stage 1

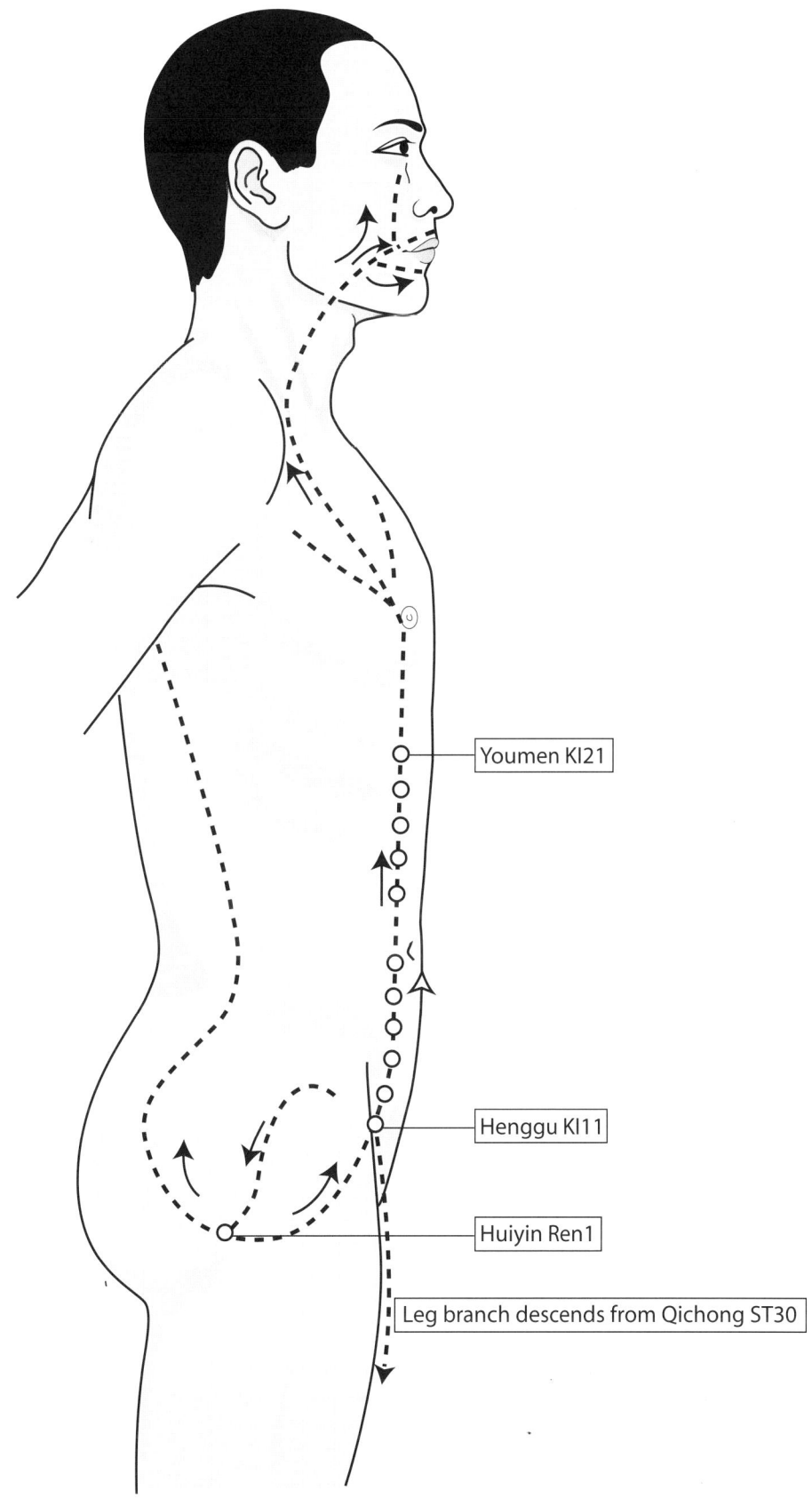

Youmen KI21

Henggu KI11

Huiyin Ren1

Leg branch descends from Qichong ST30

Figure 15.2 Chong Mai Channel — Stage 2

Dai Mai — belt

Dai Mai is the only horizontal channel in the body. It encircles the body at the waist, binding the vertical paths of the 12 main channels and in particular Chong, Ren, Kidney, Liver and Spleen Channels.

The main pathway:
- originates in the region of Zhangmen LR13
- runs obliquely downward through Daimai GB26, Wushu GB27 and Weidao GB28
- circles transversely around the waist like a belt.

The other branches:
- no internal branches.

The coalescent points are:

Daimai GB26, Wushu GB27, Weidao GB28

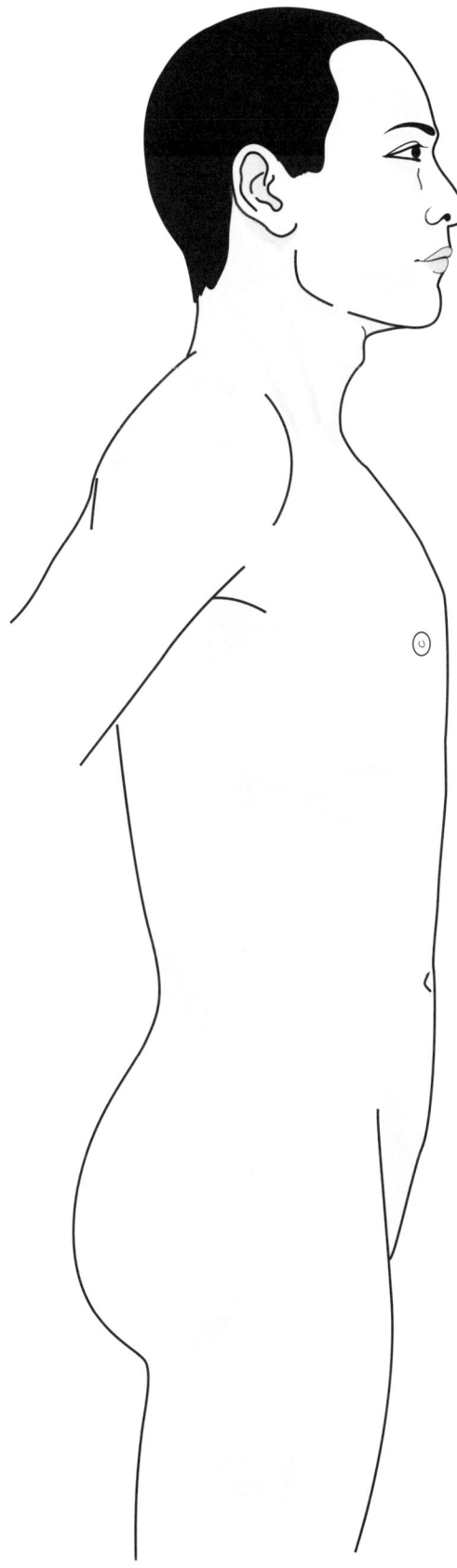

Figure 15.3 Dai Mai Channel — Stage 1

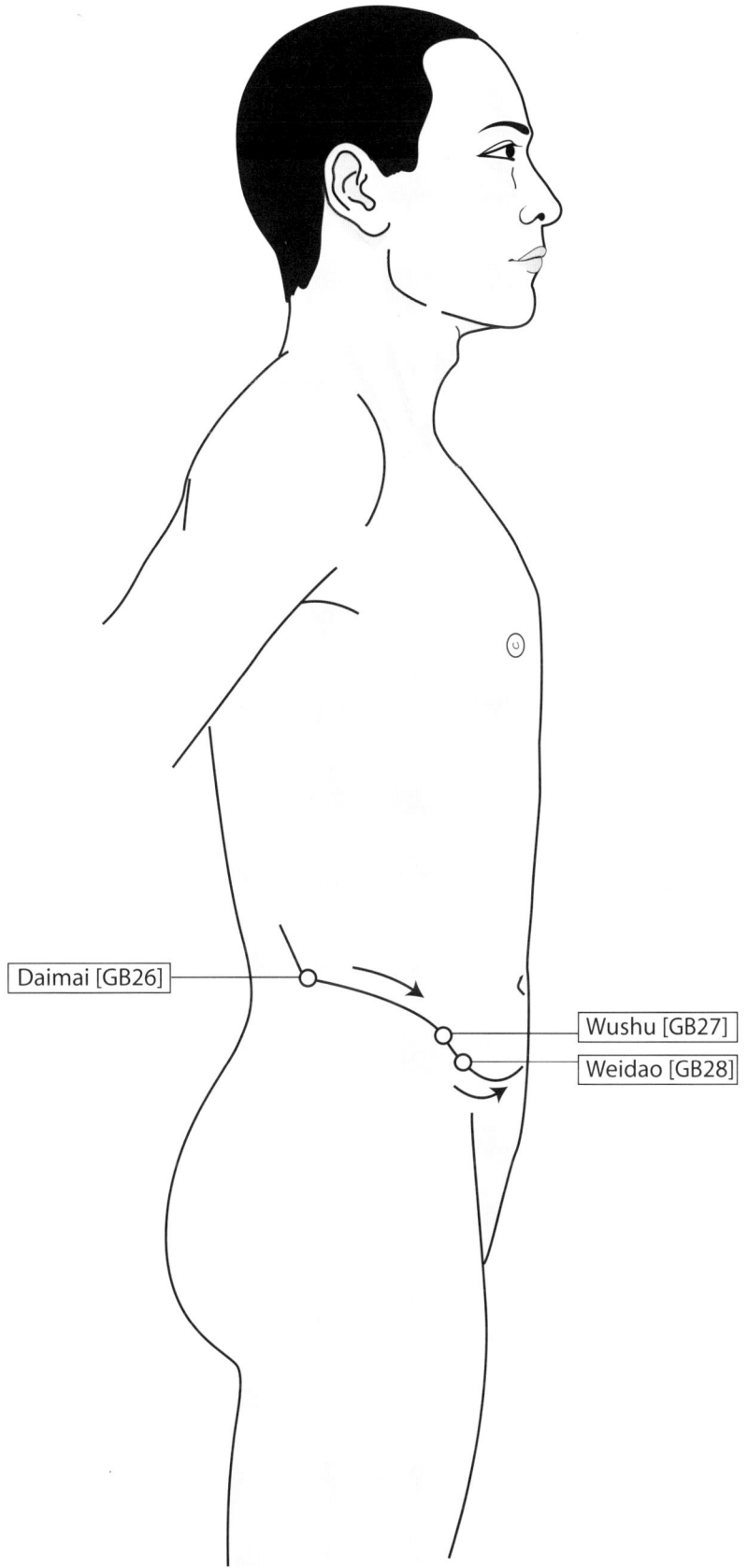

Daimai [GB26]

Wushu [GB27]

Weidao [GB28]

Figure 15.4 Dai Mai Channel — Stage 2

Yang Qiao Mai — heel/motility

Yang Qiao Mai connects the Bladder, Gall Bladder, Small Intestine, Large Intestine and Stomach Channels, and is said to dominate activity.

The main pathway:
- starts at Shenmai BL62 inferior to the lateral malleolus
- descends to Pucan BL61
- ascends along the posterior fibula following the Gall Bladder Channel to the hip
- runs upward through the lateral costal region to the posterior axillary fold
- zigzags across the top of the shoulder and runs upward along the neck to the corner of the mouth
- continues up across the cheek and alongside the nose to the inner canthus where it connects with Yin Qiao Mai at Jingming BL1
- continues upward with the Bladder Channel over the forehead
- curves across the parietal region
- descends to meet the Gall Bladder Channel at Fengchi GB20 where it enters the brain.

The other branches:
- no other branches.

The coalescent points are:

Shenmai BL62, Pucan BL61, Fuyang BL59, Femur-Juliao GB29, Naoshu SI10, Jianyu LI15, Jugu LI16, Dicang ST4, Juliao ST3, Chengqi ST1, Jingming BL1, Fengchi GB20

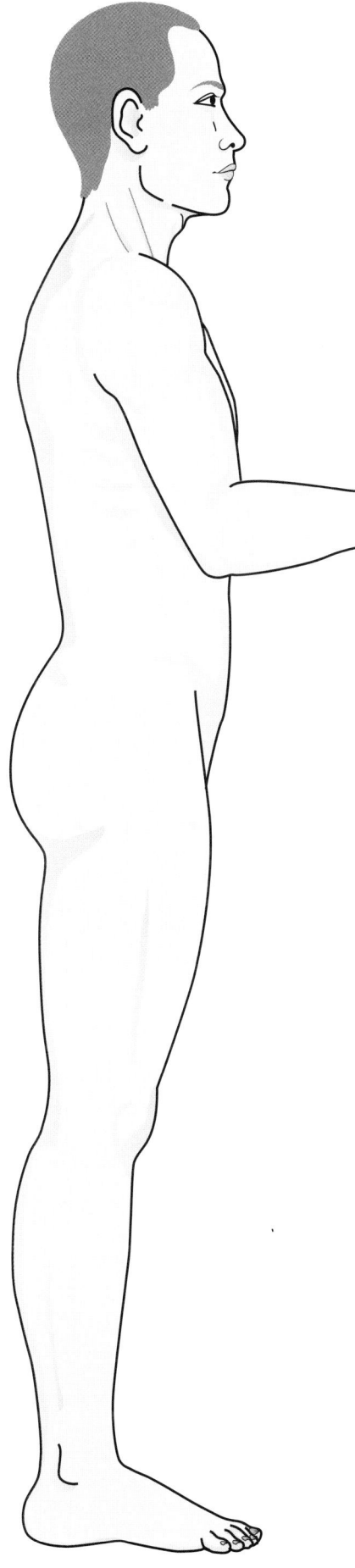

Figure 15.5 Yang Qiao Mai — Stage 1

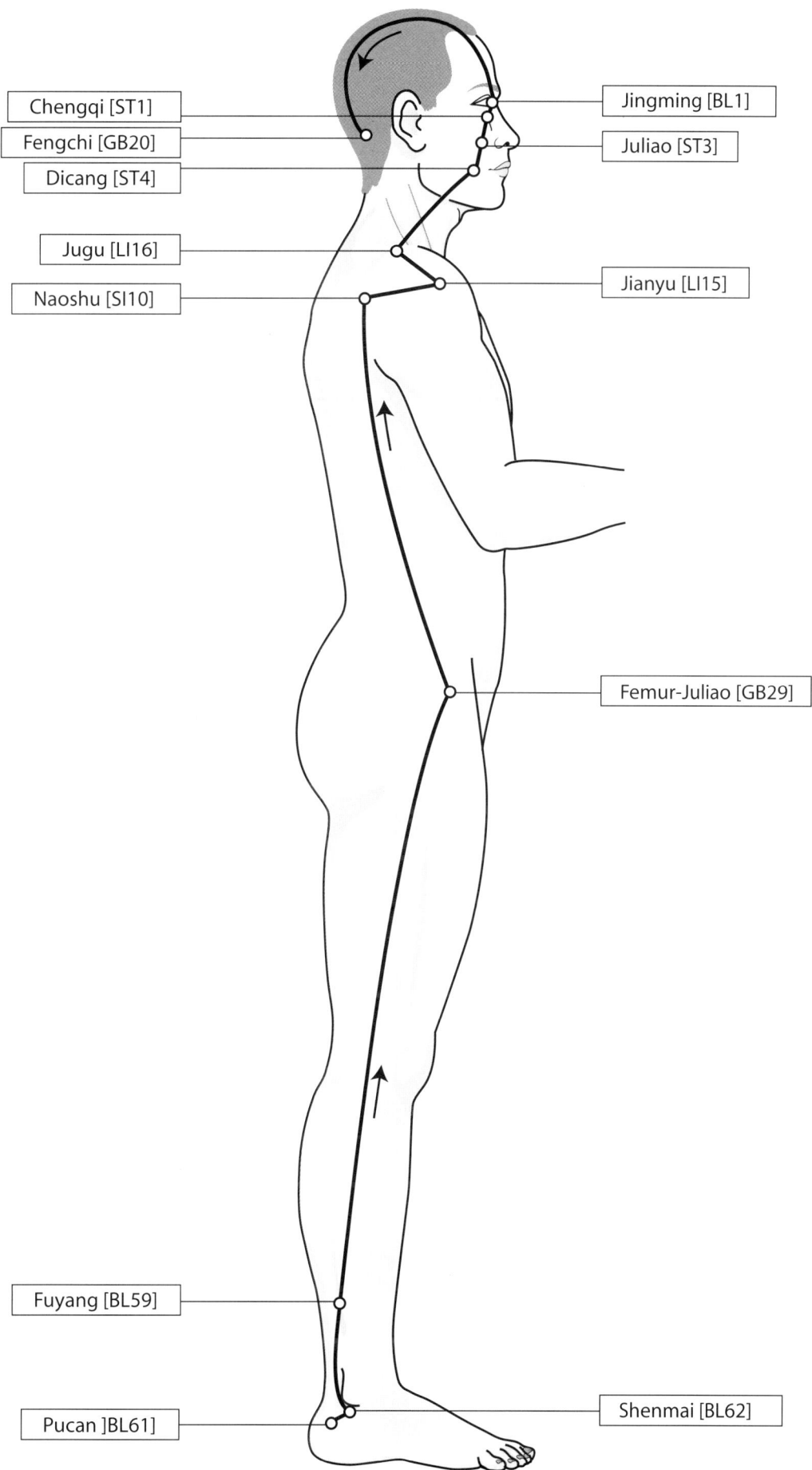

Chengqi [ST1]
Fengchi [GB20]
Dicang [ST4]
Jugu [LI16]
Naoshu [SI10]
Fuyang [BL59]
Pucan]BL61]

Jingming [BL1]
Juliao [ST3]
Jianyu [LI15]
Femur-Juliao [GB29]
Shenmai [BL62]

Figure 15.6 Yang Qiao Mai — Stage 2

Yin Qiao Mai — heel/motility

Yin Qiao Mai connects the Kidney and Bladder Channels, and is said to dominate quietness.

The main pathway:
- originates in the region of the navicular bone of the foot (close to Rangu KI2)
- passes through Zhaohai KI6 and ascends upward over the medial malleolus
- continues up the postero-medial border of the lower leg and thigh to the external genitalia
- rises through the abdomen and chest to the supraclavicular fossa
- runs upward along the throat and emerges anterior to Renying ST9
- continues over the jaw and emerges at the zygoma to reach the inner canthus of the eye where it communicates with Yang Qiao Mai and Bladder Channel at Jingming BL1 and then ascends with them to enter the brain.

The other branches:
- no other branches.

The coalescent points are:

Zhaohai KI6, Jiaoxin KI8, Jingming BL1

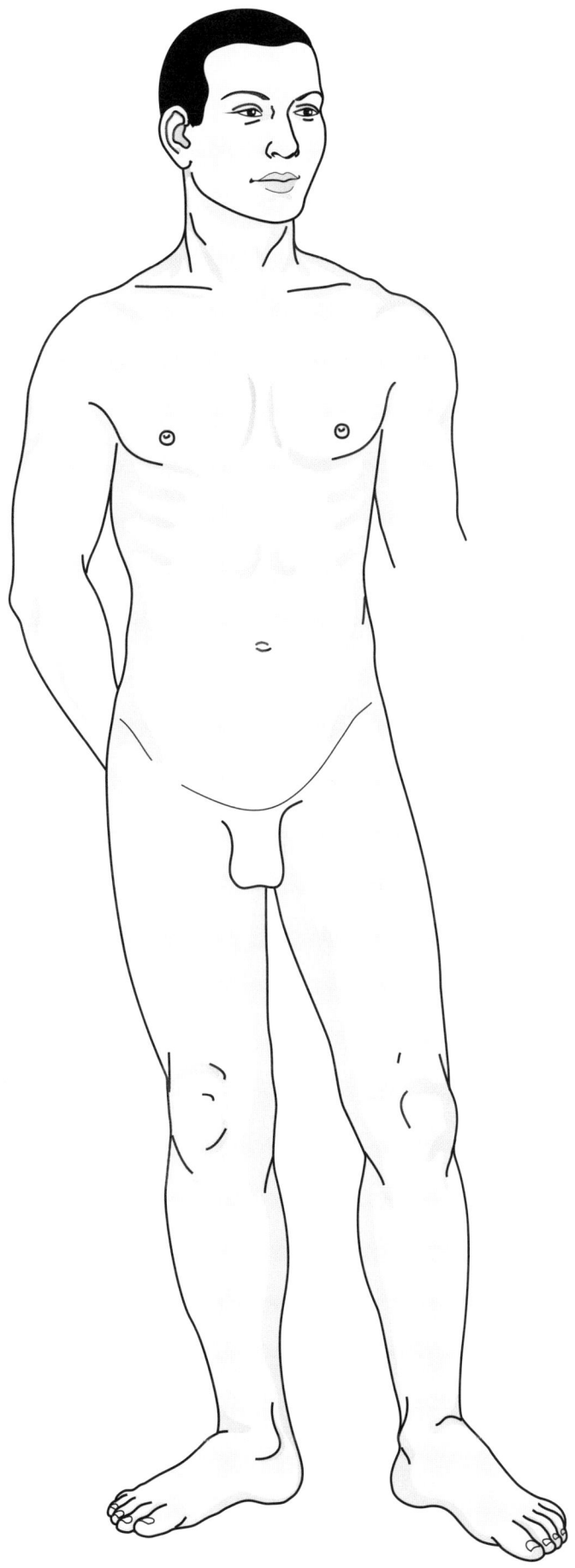

Figure 15.7 Yin Qiao Mai — Stage 1

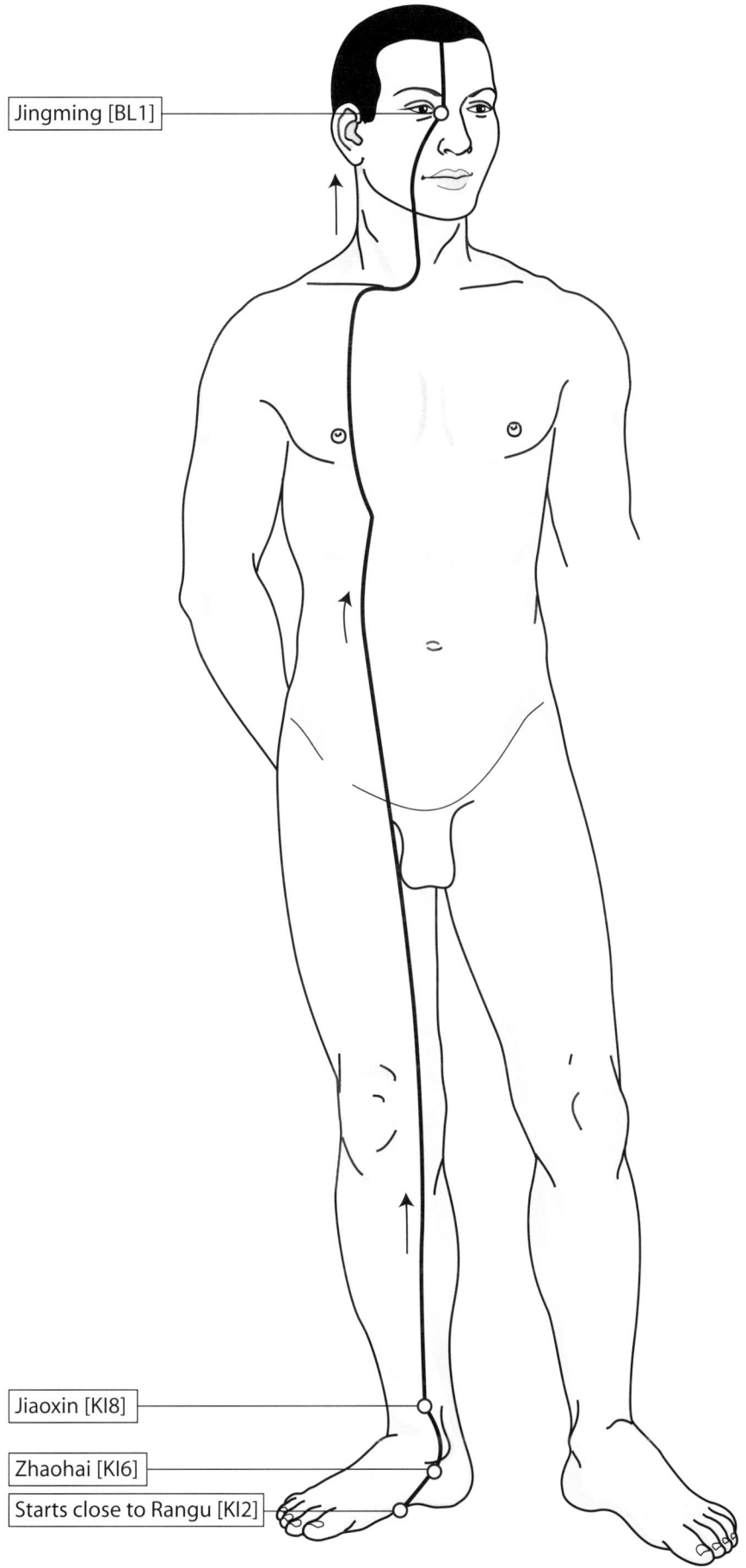

Jingming [BL1]

Jiaoxin [KI8]

Zhaohai [KI6]

Starts close to Rangu [KI2]

Figure 15.8 Yin Qiao Mai — Stage 2

Yang Wei Mai — linking

Yang Wei Mai connects the Bladder, Gall Bladder, San Jiao, Small Intestine, Stomach and Du Mai Channels, and is said to dominate the exterior of the whole body.

The main pathway:

- starts from the lateral side of the foot at Jinmen BL63

- crosses the lateral malleolus and ascends along the lateral aspect of the leg, alongside the Gall Bladder Channel, passing through the hip region

- runs up along the posterior aspect of the hypochondriac and costal regions to the posterior axillary fold

- crosses the top of the shoulder and runs up the lateral aspect of the neck and jaw

- passes anterior to the ear and continues up to the forehead at Benshen GB13

- turns downward onto the forehead at Yangbai GB14 and then runs backward across the parietal region, curving down towards the base of the occiput following the points of the Gall Bladder Channel to Fengfu Du16 and Yamen Du15.

The other branches:

- no internal branches.

The coalescent points are:

Jinmen BL63, Yangjiao GB35, Naoshu SI10, Tianliao SJ15, Jianjing GB21, Touwei ST8, Benshen GB13, Yangbai GB14, Toulinqi GB15, Muchuang GB16, Zhengying GB17, Chengling GB18, Naokong GB19, Fengchi GB20, Fengfu Du16, Yamen Du15

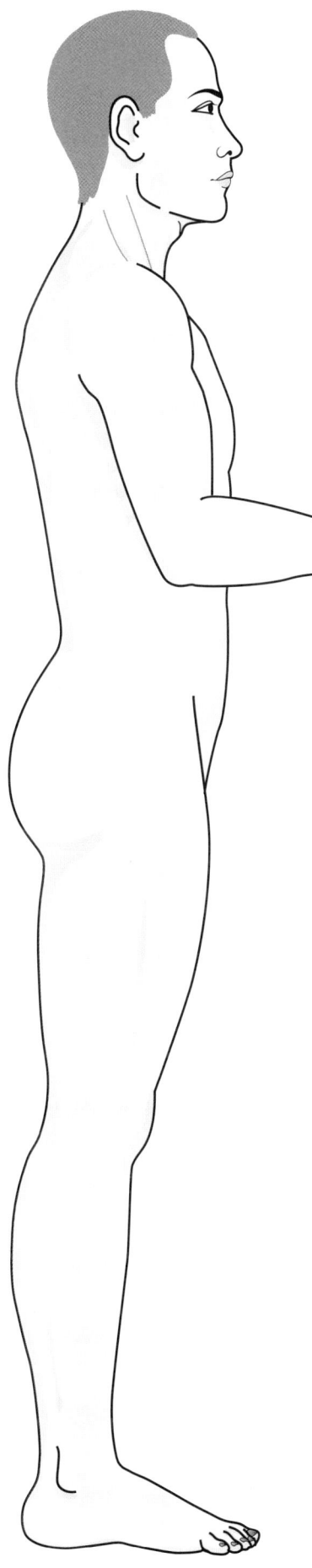

Figure 15.9 Yang Wei Mai — Stage 1

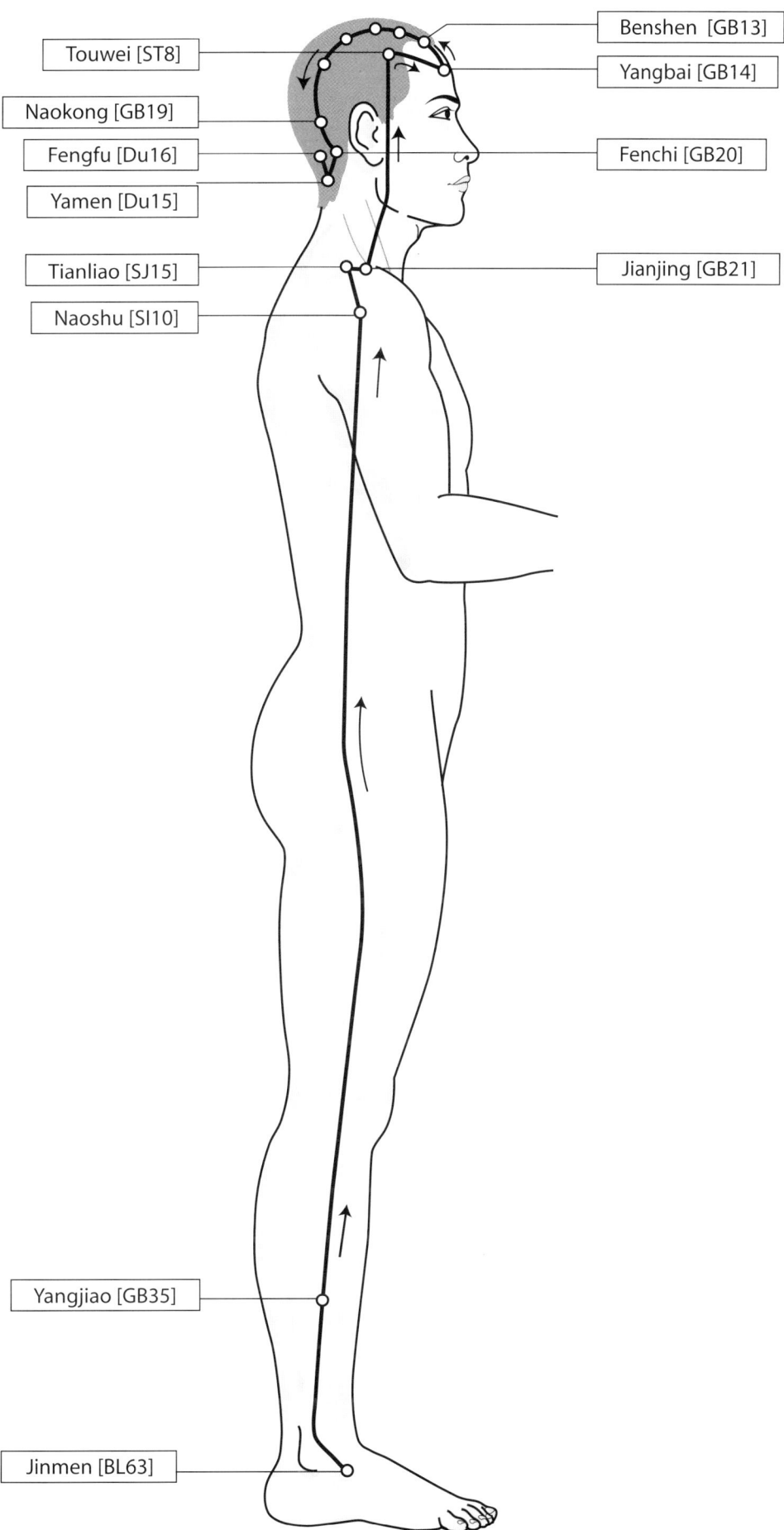

Touwei [ST8]

Naokong [GB19]

Fengfu [Du16]

Yamen [Du15]

Tianliao [SJ15]

Naoshu [SI10]

Benshen [GB13]

Yangbai [GB14]

Fenchi [GB20]

Jianjing [GB21]

Yangjiao [GB35]

Jinmen [BL63]

Figure 15.10 Yang Wei Mai — Stage 2

Yin Wei Mai — linking

Yin Wei Mai connects the Kidney, Spleen, Liver and Ren Mai Channels, and is said to dominate the interior of the whole body.

The main pathway:

- begins from the medial side of the leg at Zhubin KI9
- ascends along the medial aspect of the leg and thigh to the lower abdomen
- continues up the abdomen and crosses the chest to Qimen LR14
- runs up the throat where it connects with Ren Mai at Tiantu Ren22 and Lianquan Ren23.

The other branches:

- no internal branches.

The coalescent points are:

Zhubin KI9, Chongmen SP12, Fushe SP13, Daheng SP15, Fuai SP16, Qimen LR14, Tiantu Ren22, Lianquan Ren23

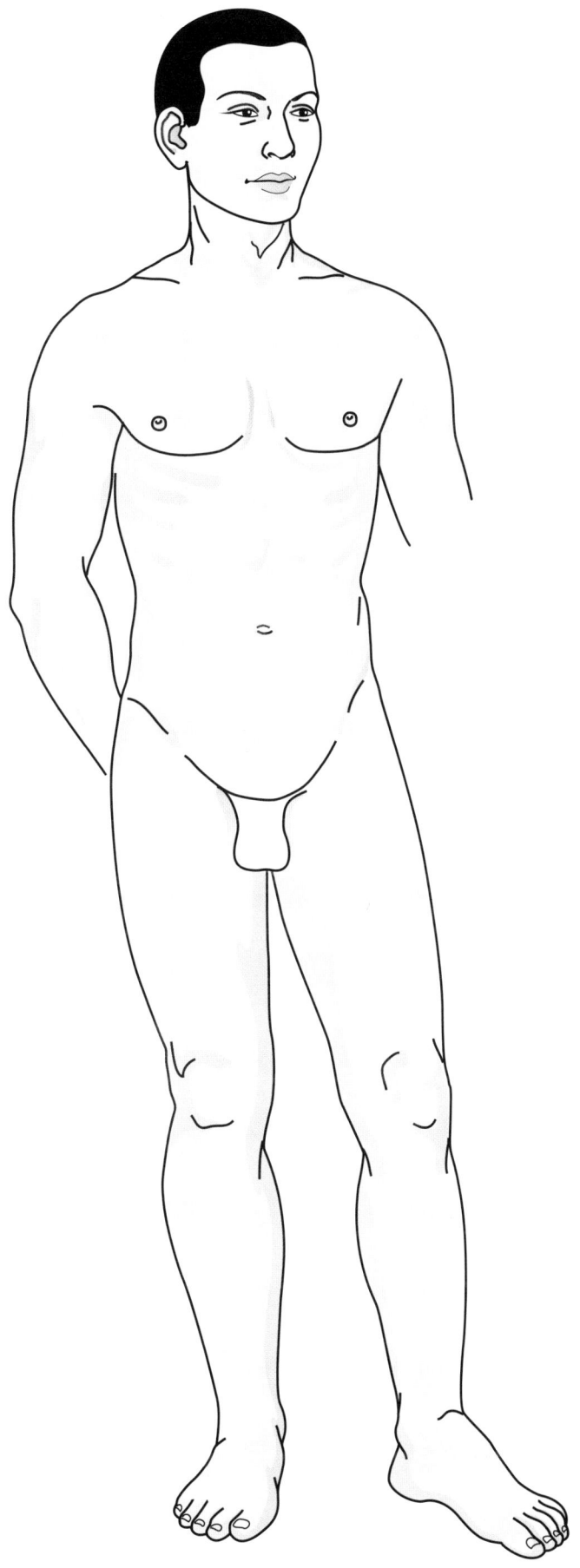

Figure 15.11 Yin Wei Mai — Stage 1

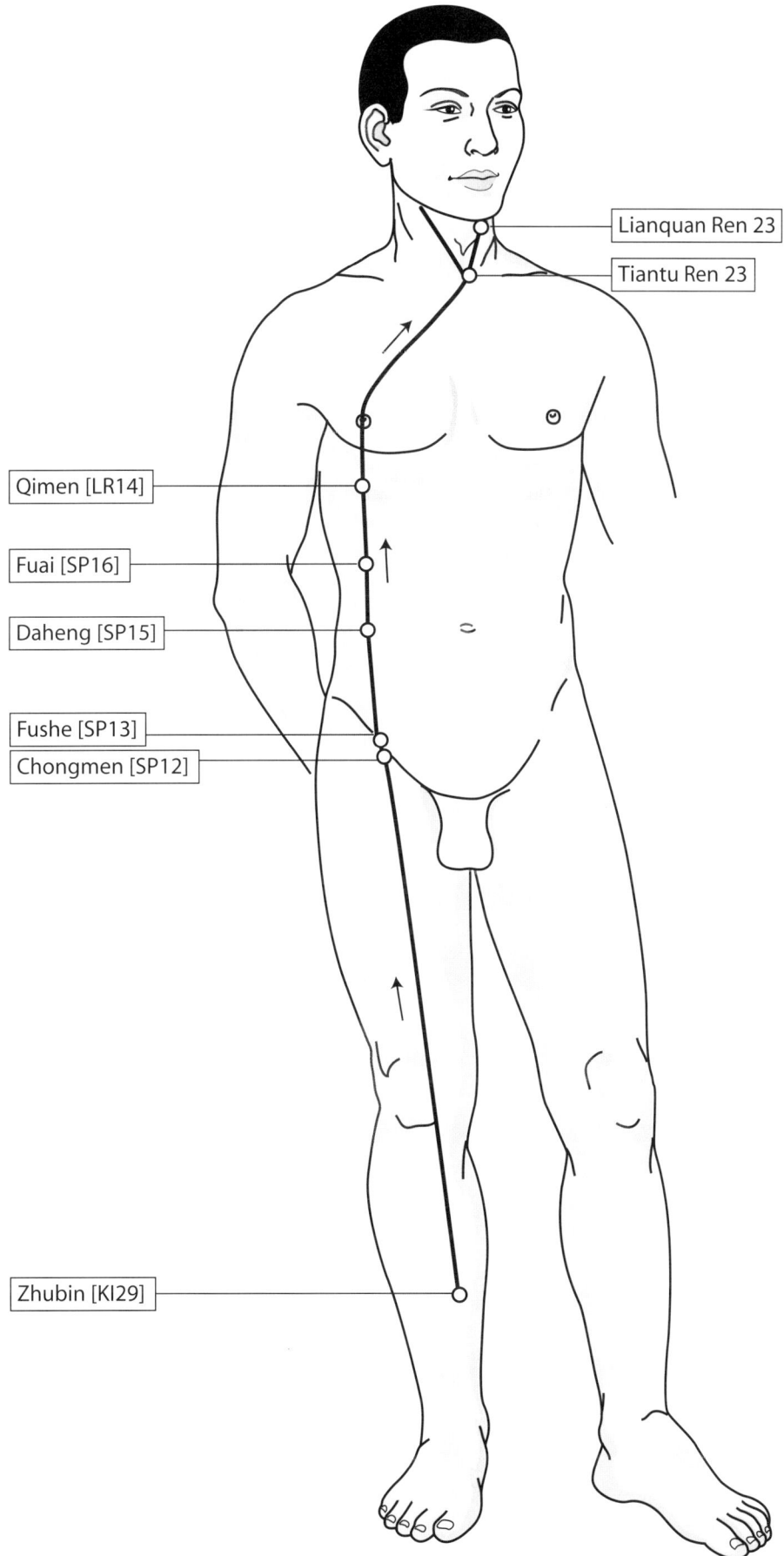

Lianquan Ren 23

Tiantu Ren 23

Qimen [LR14]

Fuai [SP16]

Daheng [SP15]

Fushe [SP13]

Chongmen [SP12]

Zhubin [KI29]

Figure 15.12 Yin Wei Mai — Stage 2

THE OTHER SIX EXTRAORDINARY VESSELS — CASE STUDIES

One of the most important clinical uses of the extraordinary vessels is their use in pairs as coupled channels, the function of one supplementing the function of another (see table below).

Each pair is activated by using the confluent or master points of its two channels, for example:

The Ren Mai and Yin Qiao Mai pair is activated by using Lieque LU7 with Zhaohai KI6, the appropriate confluent points.

Using the table below, answer the following clinical cases using the master points on the extraordinary vessels and any additional points you feel are relevant.

Keep it simple and in harmony.

EIGHT EXTRAORDINARY VESSELS (IN COUPLED PAIRS)			
Channels (pairs)	Main associated channels	Main associated organs	Master point
Ren Mai Yin Qiao Mai	Ren, KI, LU	KI, LU	LU7 Lieque KI6 Zhaohai
Du Mai Yang Qiao Mai	Du, BL, SI	KI, HT, LR	SI3 Houxi BL62 Shenmai
Chong Mai Yin Wei Mai	KI, SP, PC	KI, SP, HT	SP4 Gongsun PC6 Neiguan
Dai Mai Yang Wei Mai	GB, SJ, LR	GB, LR	GB41 Zulinqqi SJ5 Waiguan

1 **A person with deficient spleen qi, abdominal distension, tiredness, loose stool, poor appetite.**

2 **A person with hyperactive liver yang headache, spinal stiffness and deficient kidney qi.**

3 **A person with deficient heart qi and blood, as well as palpitations and insomnia.**

4 **A person with asthma, cough, difficulty speaking (tension of vocal cords with fear).**

5 **A person with occipital headaches, dizziness, neck and shoulder problems, ear and eye problems.**

The extra points (20)

These points are numbered according to the notation in *Chinese Acupuncture and Moxibustion* (Cheng 1987, pp 231–43). The notation from *A Manual of Acupuncture* is also given for reference (Deadman et al 2006, pp 565–85).

The extra points (also known as 'extraordinary points') are experiential points with specific names and locations that do not belong to the 12 primary channels, Ren Mai or Du Mai, although some of them lie on their courses.

Scattered over the body, these points are still related to the channel system; for example, Lanwei Ex37 is related to the Stomach Channel of Foot Yangming, and Yintang Ex1 to the Du Channel.

Historically there is a great range in the number of extra points (20–1500) published in the last few decades. Some of the points on the primary channels developed from extra points; for example, Gaohuang BL43, Meichong BL3.

Clinically these points augment the 'regular' points on the 12 primary channels and are effective in the treatment of specific disorders; for example, Yaotongxue Ex29 is a commonly used point for acute lumbar strain.

WHO number	Pinyin	Name	Deadman et al
Ex1	**Taiyang**	Supreme Yang	M-HN-9
Ex2	**Yintang**	Hall of Impression	M-HN-3
Ex4	**Erjian**	Tip of the Ear	M-HN-10
Ex5	**Yuyao**	Fish Waist	M-HN-6
Ex6	**Sishencong**	Four Alert Spirit	M-HN-1
Ex10	**Bitong**	Penetrating the Nose	M-HN-14
Ex13	**Anmian**	Peaceful Sleep	M-HN-54
Ex14	**Dingchuan**	Calm Dyspnoea	M-BW-1
Ex15	**Huatuojiaji**	Hua Tuo's Paravertebral Points	M-BW-35
Ex16	**Bailao**	Hundred Taxations	M-HN-30
Ex18	**Shiqizhui(xia)**	Below the Seventeenth Vertebra	M-BW-25
Ex21	**Yaoyan**	Lumbar Eyes	M-BW-24
Ex27	**Baxie**	Eight Pathogens	M-UE-22
Ex28	**Luozhen**	Stiff Neck	M-UE-24
Ex29	**Yaotongxue**	Lumbar Point Pain	N-UE-19
Ex36	**Xiyan (Neixiyan)**	Eyes of the Knee	MN-LE-16
Ex37	**Lanwei(xue)**	Appendix Point	M-LE-13
Ex38	**Heding**	Crane's Summit	M-LE-27
Ex39	**Dannangxue**	Gall Bladder Point	M-LE-23
Ex40	**Bafeng**	Eight Winds	M-LE-8

Note: The 20 points listed are those the author has found most useful in clinical practice. However, different teaching programs will place an emphasis on different groups of points. These points are distributed all over the body and can be added to any existing diagrams.

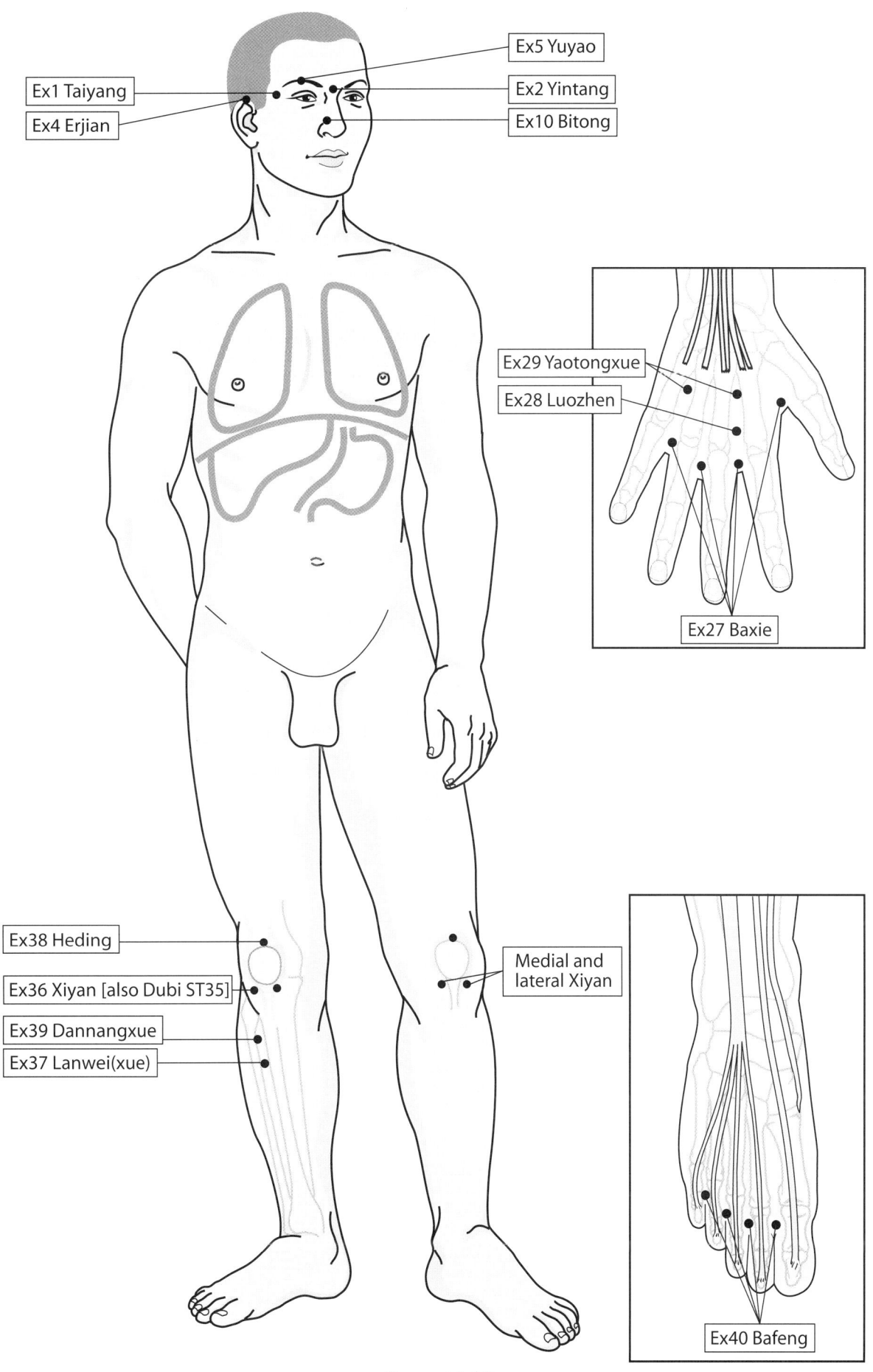

Ex5 Yuyao

Ex1 Taiyang

Ex4 Erjian

Ex2 Yintang

Ex10 Bitong

Ex29 Yaotongxue

Ex28 Luozhen

Ex27 Baxie

Ex38 Heding

Ex36 Xiyan [also Dubi ST35]

Ex39 Dannangxue

Ex37 Lanwei(xue)

Medial and lateral Xiyan

Ex40 Bafeng

Figure 15.13

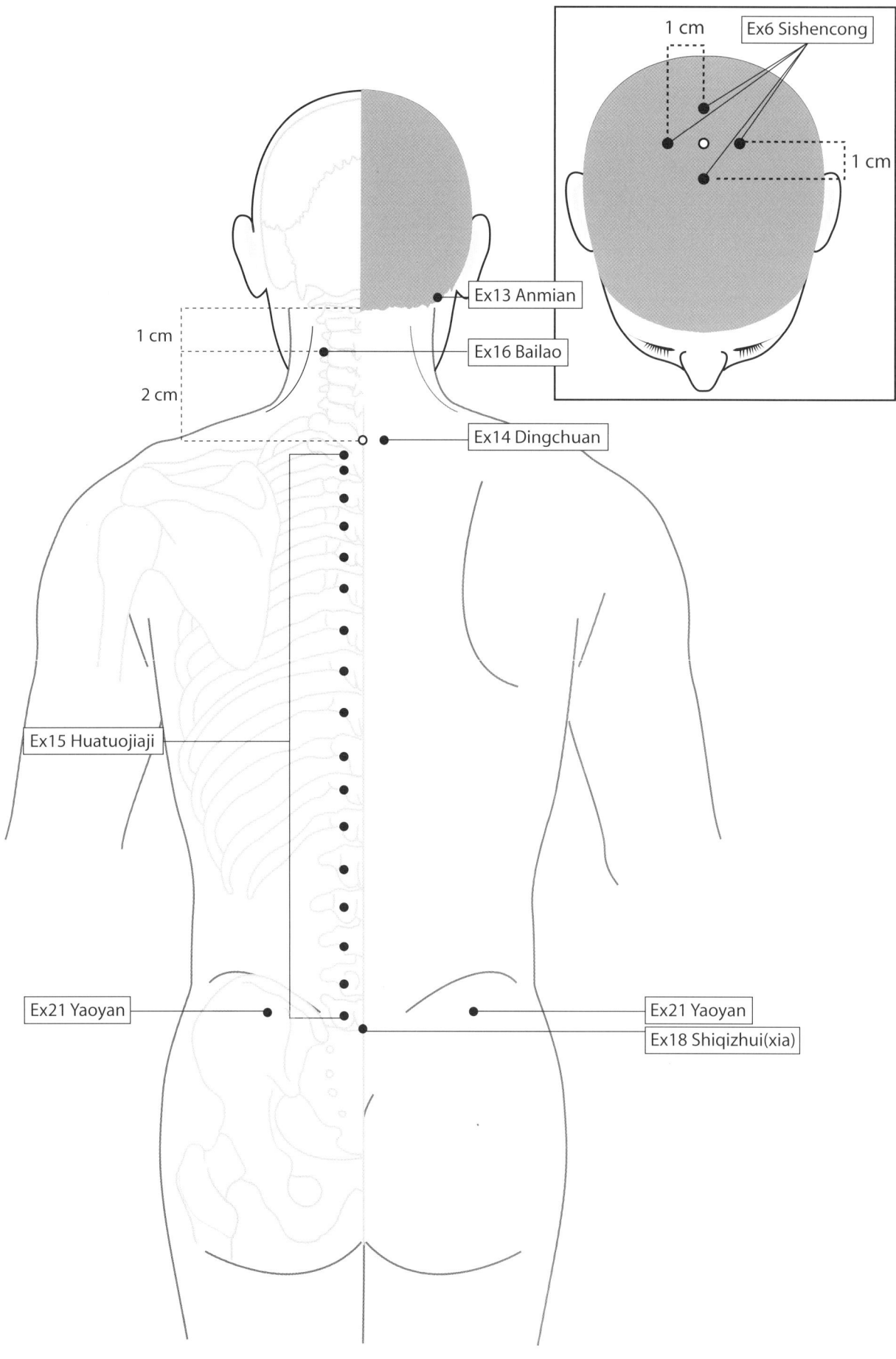

1 cm

Ex6 Sishencong

1 cm

Ex13 Anmian

1 cm

Ex16 Bailao

2 cm

Ex14 Dingchuan

Ex15 Huatuojiaji

Ex21 Yaoyan

Ex21 Yaoyan

Ex18 Shiqizhui(xia)

Figure 15.14

ANATOMICAL APPENDIX

Chinese medicine uses living surface anatomy as a fundamental method of locating acupuncture points on the twelve primary channels, and Ren Mai and Du Mai.

The Chinese were great observers of nature and the human body, and likened the Jing Mai to the rivers of China flowing over the landscape providing nourishment, connection and transport.

So, the landscape of the body provides a living map and guides the flows of the channels (like rivers) through the depressions and around the prominences on the body — for example Yanglingquan (GB34) is in the depression anterior and inferior to the head of the fibula, Quchi (LI11) is the depression at the lateral end of the cubital crease when the elbow is flexed.

There are three methods for locating points:

1. surface anatomical landmarks

2. proportional measurement (the length between two joints)

3. hand (*cun*) measurement.

These methods are often used in combination.

It is therefore important and relevant to have an understanding of basic human anatomy, and its component parts, in order to locate points accurately.

This is a patient safety issue. Students and practitioners have a responsibility to make careful observation and palpation of the areas to be needled so that underlying structures, such as major arteries, veins, nerves and organs, are not damaged.

Every effort has been made to show the channel flows in this book as anatomically precise as possible on a two-dimensional image.

Use the anatomical information from this appendix, and from your own anatomy texts, to draw in any anatomical markers you need — for example, bones, tendons, ligaments, nerves, arteries, veins and so forth. This will help you to reinforce your learning of channel flows and point locations.

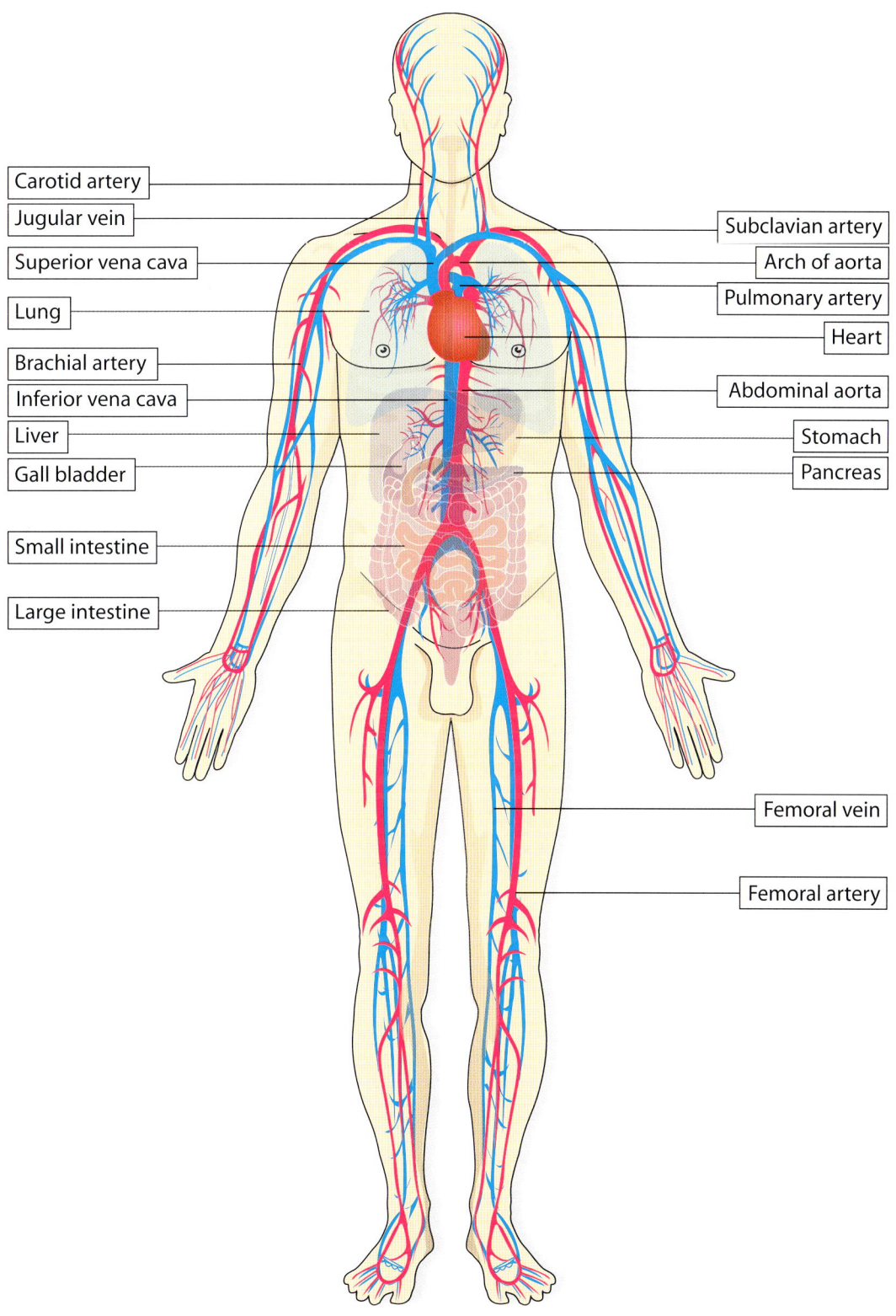

Carotid artery	Subclavian artery
Jugular vein	Arch of aorta
Superior vena cava	Pulmonary artery
Lung	Heart
Brachial artery	Abdominal aorta
Inferior vena cava	Stomach
Liver	Pancreas
Gall bladder	
Small intestine	
Large intestine	
	Femoral vein
	Femoral artery

Circulatory System

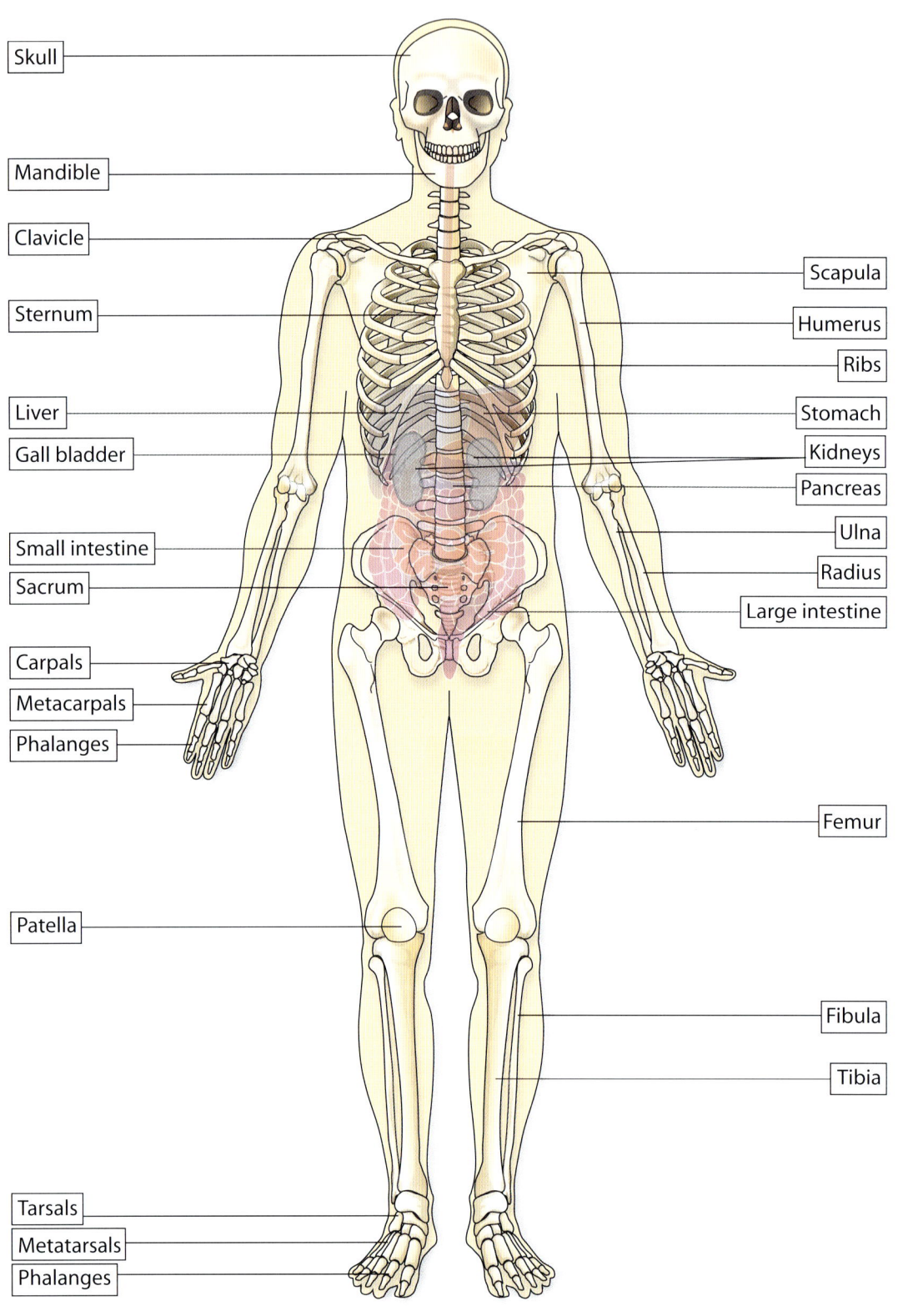

Skull

Mandible

Clavicle

Sternum

Liver

Gall bladder

Small intestine

Sacrum

Carpals

Metacarpals

Phalanges

Patella

Tarsals

Metatarsals

Phalanges

Scapula

Humerus

Ribs

Stomach

Kidneys

Pancreas

Ulna

Radius

Large intestine

Femur

Fibula

Tibia

Skeleton (front)

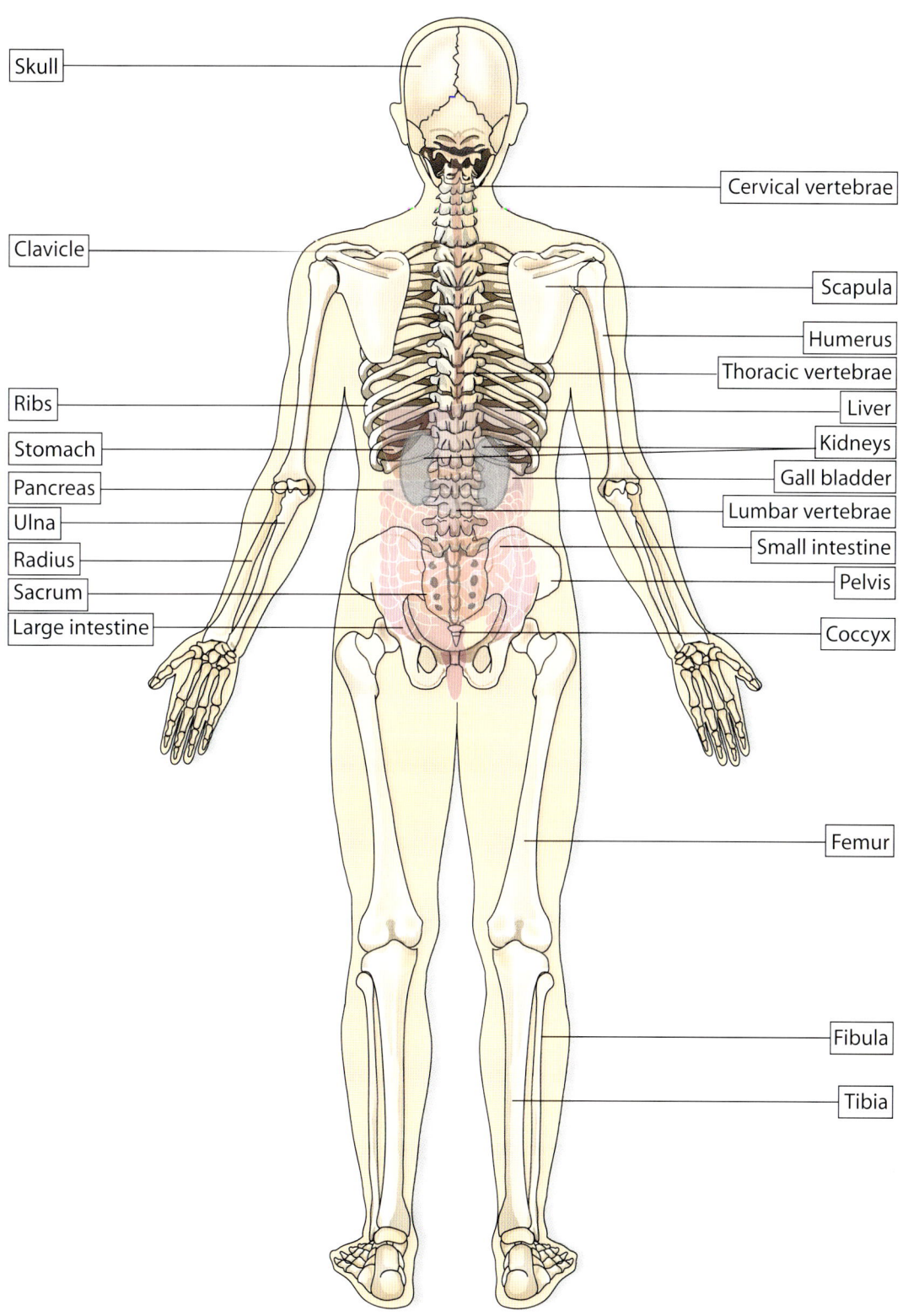

Skull

Cervical vertebrae

Clavicle

Scapula

Humerus

Thoracic vertebrae

Ribs

Liver

Stomach

Kidneys

Pancreas

Gall bladder

Ulna

Lumbar vertebrae

Radius

Small intestine

Sacrum

Pelvis

Large intestine

Coccyx

Femur

Fibula

Tibia

Skeleton (back)

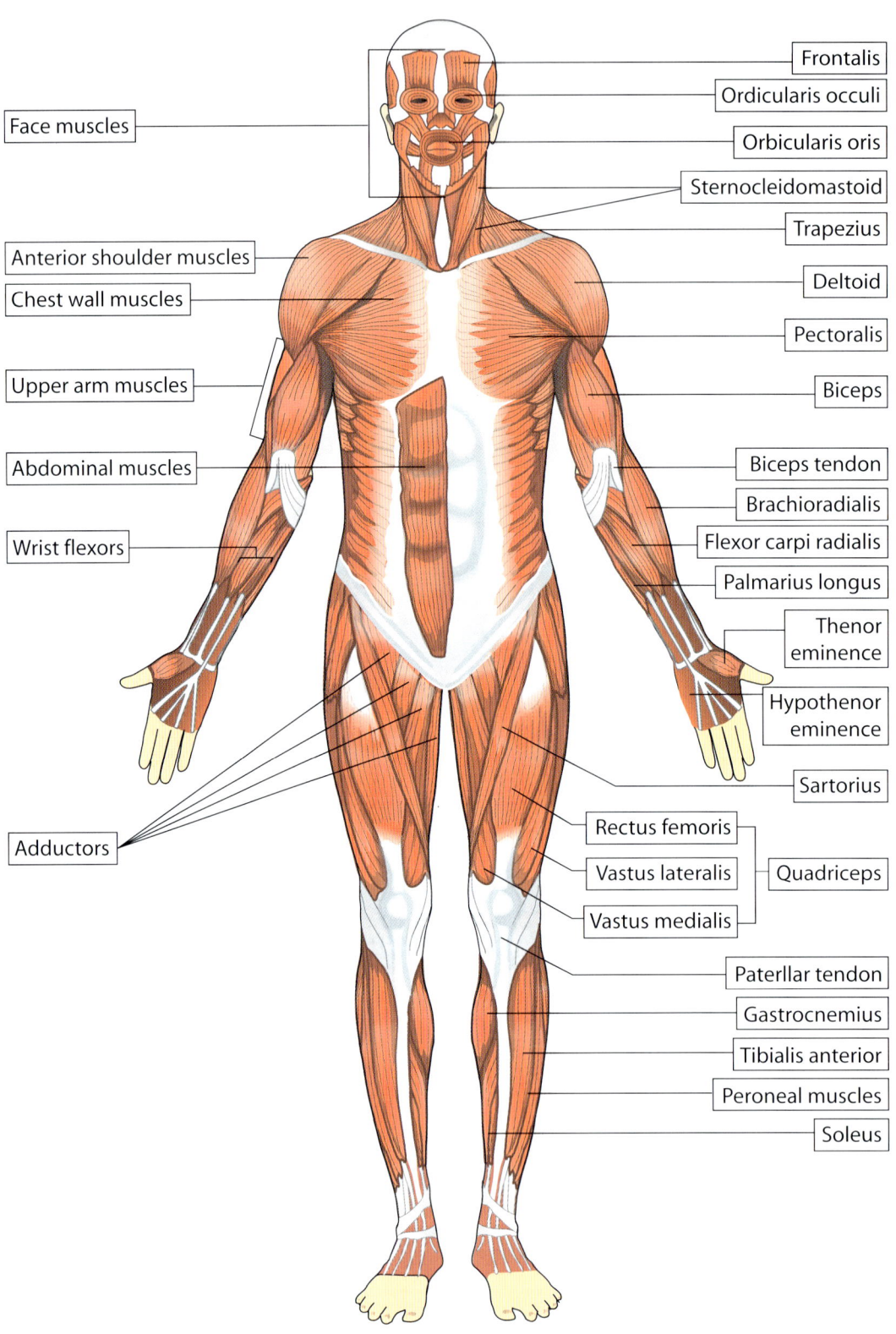

Face muscles

Anterior shoulder muscles

Chest wall muscles

Upper arm muscles

Abdominal muscles

Wrist flexors

Adductors

Frontalis

Ordicularis occuli

Orbicularis oris

Sternocleidomastoid

Trapezius

Deltoid

Pectoralis

Biceps

Biceps tendon

Brachioradialis

Flexor carpi radialis

Palmarius longus

Thenor eminence

Hypothenor eminence

Sartorius

Rectus femoris

Vastus lateralis

Vastus medialis

Quadriceps

Paterllar tendon

Gastrocnemius

Tibialis anterior

Peroneal muscles

Soleus

Musculature (front)

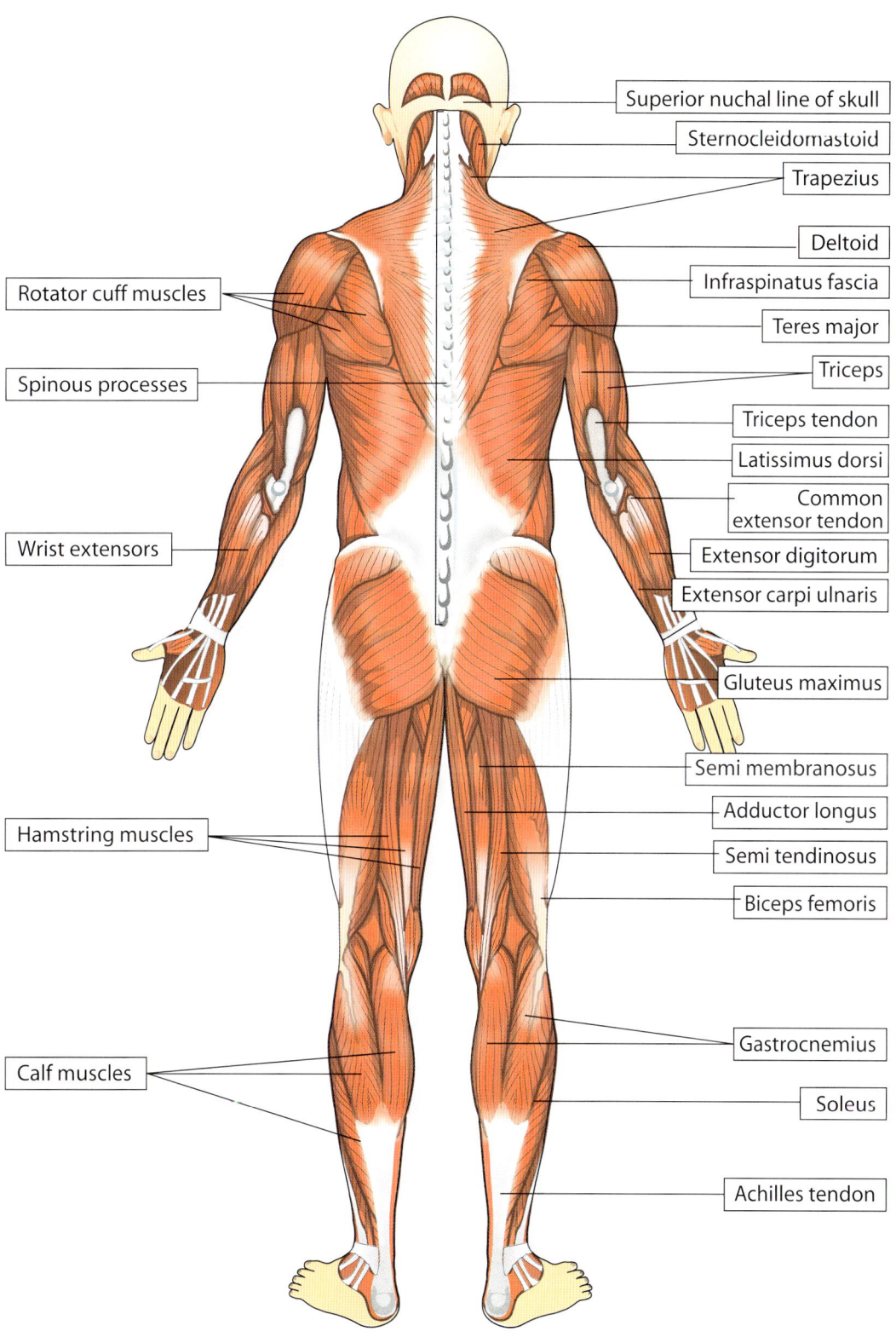

Superior nuchal line of skull

Sternocleidomastoid

Trapezius

Deltoid

Infraspinatus fascia

Teres major

Triceps

Triceps tendon

Latissimus dorsi

Common extensor tendon

Extensor digitorum

Extensor carpi ulnaris

Gluteus maximus

Semi membranosus

Adductor longus

Semi tendinosus

Biceps femoris

Gastrocnemius

Soleus

Achilles tendon

Rotator cuff muscles

Spinous processes

Wrist extensors

Hamstring muscles

Calf muscles

Musculature (back)

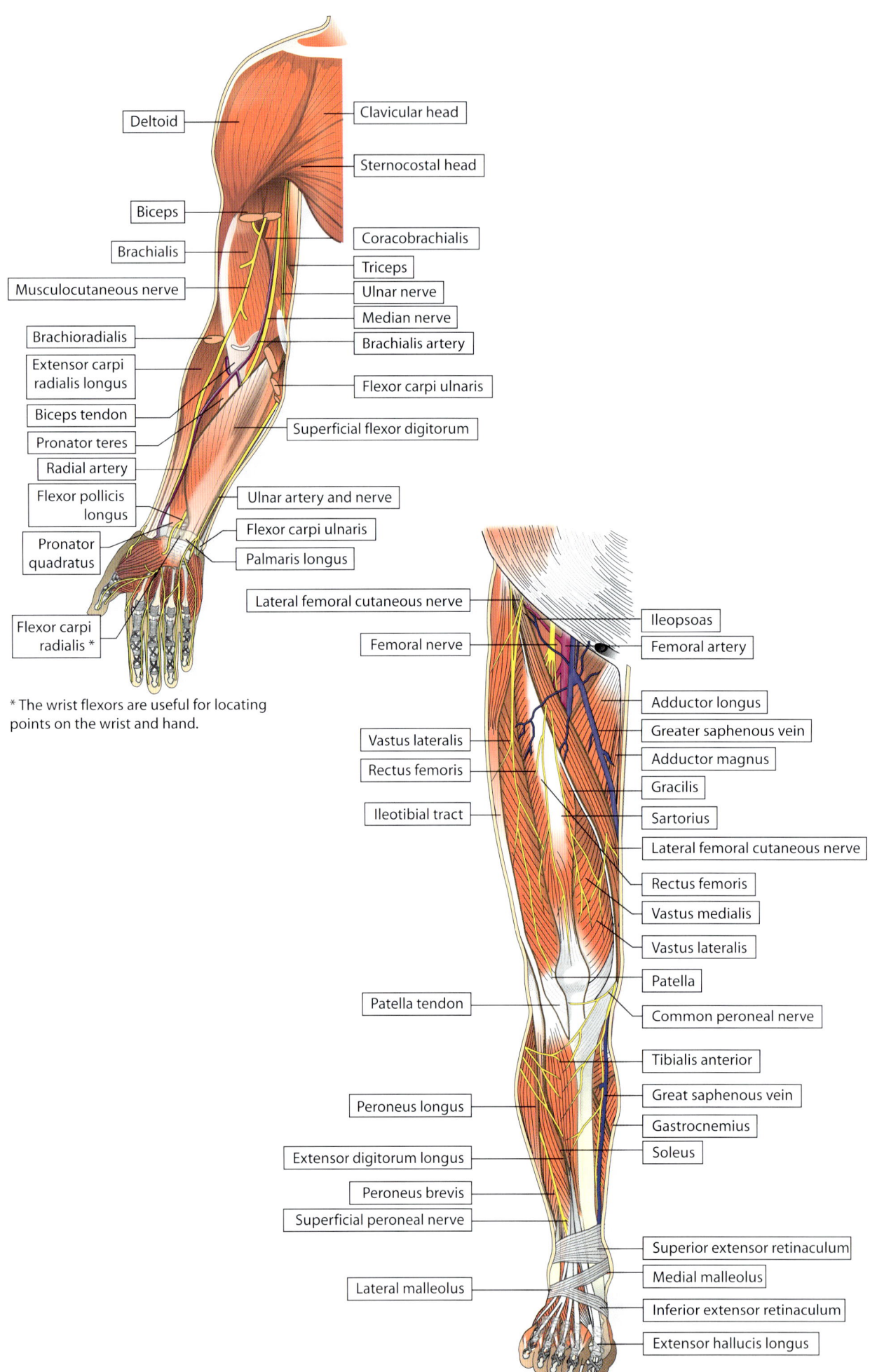

Deltoid

Clavicular head

Sternocostal head

Biceps

Coracobrachialis

Brachialis

Triceps

Musculocutaneous nerve

Ulnar nerve

Median nerve

Brachioradialis

Brachialis artery

Extensor carpi
radialis longus

Biceps tendon

Flexor carpi ulnaris

Pronator teres

Superficial flexor digitorum

Radial artery

Flexor pollicis
longus

Ulnar artery and nerve

Pronator
quadratus

Flexor carpi ulnaris

Palmaris longus

Flexor carpi
radialis *

Lateral femoral cutaneous nerve

Ileopsoas

Femoral nerve

Femoral artery

Adductor longus

Greater saphenous vein

Vastus lateralis

Adductor magnus

Rectus femoris

Gracilis

Ileotibial tract

Sartorius

Lateral femoral cutaneous nerve

Rectus femoris

Vastus medialis

Vastus lateralis

Patella

Patella tendon

Common peroneal nerve

Tibialis anterior

Great saphenous vein

Peroneus longus

Gastrocnemius

Extensor digitorum longus

Soleus

Peroneus brevis

Superficial peroneal nerve

Superior extensor retinaculum

Medial malleolus

Inferior extensor retinaculum

Lateral malleolus

Extensor hallucis longus

* The wrist flexors are useful for locating
points on the wrist and hand.

Upper Limb (Medial layer) and Lower Limb (Superficial Layer), front

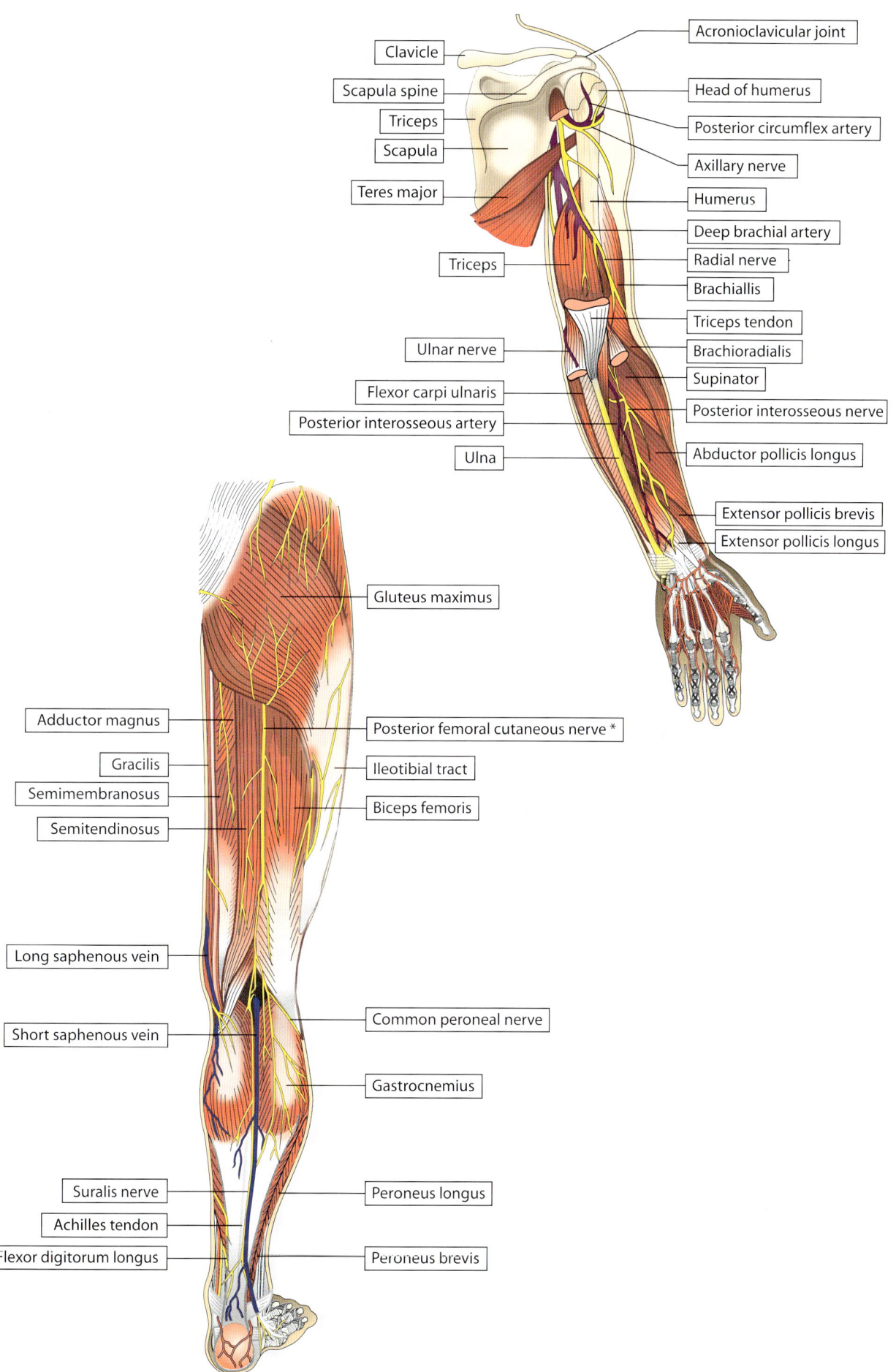

Clavicle

Acronioclavicular joint

Scapula spine

Head of humerus

Triceps

Posterior circumflex artery

Scapula

Axillary nerve

Teres major

Humerus

Deep brachial artery

Triceps

Radial nerve

Brachiallis

Triceps tendon

Ulnar nerve

Brachioradialis

Flexor carpi ulnaris

Supinator

Posterior interosseous artery

Posterior interosseous nerve

Ulna

Abductor pollicis longus

Extensor pollicis brevis

Extensor pollicis longus

Gluteus maximus

Adductor magnus

Posterior femoral cutaneous nerve *

Gracilis

Ileotibial tract

Semimembranosus

Biceps femoris

Semitendinosus

Long saphenous vein

Short saphenous vein

Common peroneal nerve

Gastrocnemius

Suralis nerve

Peroneus longus

Achilles tendon

Flexor digitorum longus

Peroneus brevis

* at a deeper layer the sciatic nerve runs down the back of the leg to the popliteal fossa where it branches into the tibial ad common peroneal nerves.

Upper Limb (Medial layer) and Lower Limb (Superficial Layer), back

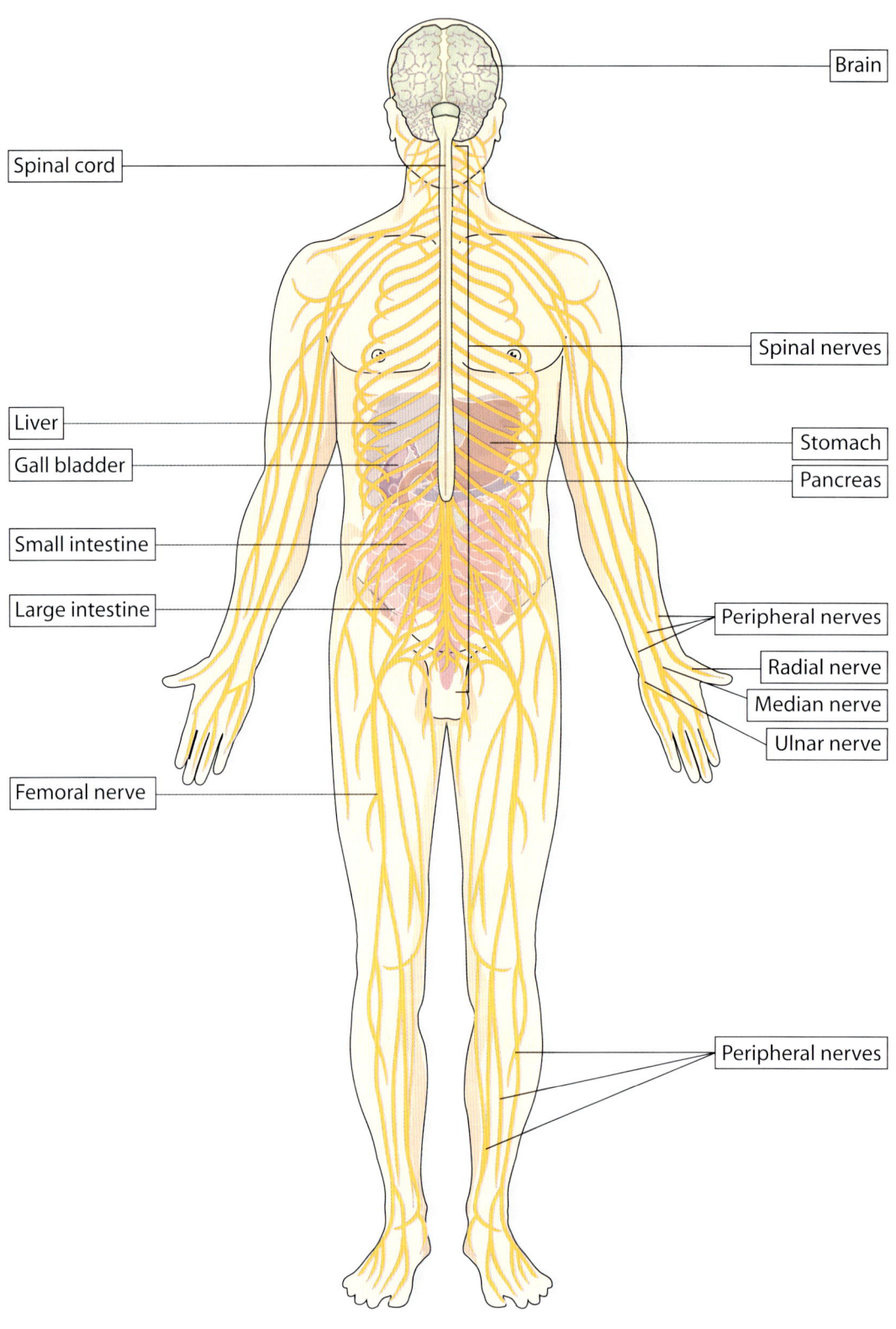

Brain

Spinal cord

Spinal nerves

Liver

Stomach

Gall bladder

Pancreas

Small intestine

Large intestine

Peripheral nerves

Radial nerve

Median nerve

Ulnar nerve

Femoral nerve

Peripheral nerves

Nervous system

ANSWERS TO CASE STUDIES

Guidelines to answers

This exercise is about learning to combine points into a simple, effective prescription; it is not necessary to use all the points listed at any one time.

Therefore the case study answers offer a selection of points from which a treatment prescription can be made.

Please note: where 'normal' appears in the answers below, this indicates 'normal' for that person.

Chapter 1 The Lung Channel — Miss MP, 26 year old receptionist

1 external

2 **a** cold

    b wind

    c acute

3 –

4 initially 'normal' rate and rhythm, with time will become tense and superficial

5 may be 'normal' initially, a thin white coating may be present

6 **ben** — drastic climatic changes and weak defensive qi (wei qi)

    biao — acute invasion by external wind and cold

7 eliminate wind, disperse cold, release the exterior syndrome by promoting sweating, stop cough, strengthen wei qi and promote lung's dispersing and descending function of qi and jin ye

8 **Zhongfu LU1**, front-mu point of lung — disperses heat in lung, direct action on lung

    Chize LU5, he-sea point, water point — makes lung qi descend

    Kongzui LU6, xi-cleft point — use in acute situations for diseases of lung and blood, causes lung qi to descend

    Lieque LU7, luo-connecting point, master point of Ren Mai — strengthens dispersing and descending functions of lung, releases the exterior, disperses wind and cold, circulates the wei qi, treats nasal obstruction and runny nose

    Taiyuan LU9, yuan-source point, shu-stream point, influential point of vessels — strengthens lung qi and transforms phlegm, promotes the descending function of lung

Chapter 2 The Large Intestine Channel — Mr DC, 24 year old rugby player

1 external

2 **a** hot

    b –

c acute — this is an acute injury with damage to the rotator cuff muscles, tendons and ligaments following trauma. Qi and blood stasis will occur in the local area and affected channels (LU, LI, SI, SJ, GB). Recovery may be complicated by an underlying blood deficiency failing to nourish tendons and ligaments or external pathogen obstruction (painful Bi syndrome).

3 –

4 normal or slightly fast rate, regular, deep, strong

5 in the early stages of acute injury the tongue may be normal

6 **ben** — if the injury is recurrent it will indicate underlying patterns of imbalance such as liver blood deficiency

biao — injury to muscle, tendon and ligament following trauma

7 decrease pain and restore range of movement by clearing local qi stagnation and blood stasis, restore normal flows of qi and blood in the affected channels, nourish blood and correct any underlying patterns of imbalance

8 **Hegu LI4**, yuan-source point — powerful calming and antispasmodic action, treats pain along the channel, treats Bi syndrome

Wenliu LI7, xi-cleft point — treats acute conditions, pain and aching in the shoulder and arm

Shousanli LI10 — activates the channel and relieves pain, indicated for pain and immobility of the shoulder, alternate with Quchi LI11

Quchi LI11, he-sea point, earth point — activates the channel and relieves pain, treats Bi syndrome

Binao LI14 — useful when pain radiates down from shoulder

Jianyu LI15, meeting point with Yang Qiao Mai — major point for the treatment of shoulder and upper arm pain, eliminates wind, damp, regulates qi and blood, reduces pain

Jugu LI16 — alleviates pain along the channel and benefits the shoulder joint, frequently used with LI15

Zhongfu LU1, front-mu point (LU) — use as local point for anterior joint pain or biceps tendon pain

Chize LU5, he-sea point, water point (LU) — useful for anterior shoulder pain

Taiyuan LU9, yuan-source point, shu-stream point (LU), influential point of vessels — treats pain along the Lung Channel, including the shoulder

Note: This case generated lots of discussion in class. Some students argued that accidents only happen when there is underlying deficiency (such as blood xu) which allows the external force to cause injury, with subsequent damage to local channels, qi and blood. These students argued for an internal disorder, hot, with blood deficiency (xu) and stagnant qi and blood (shi).

Chapter 3 The Stomach Channel — Mr NL, 65 year old retired accountant

1 internal

2 –

3 a both; deficient — stomach qi fails to descend (failure to send down the turbid qi leading to retention of food in the stomach); excess — rebellious stomach qi

b heat

c stomach, large intestine, lung

d Stomach, Large Intestine and Lung Channels

4 rate may be increased, regular, slippery and full, strong

5 tongue body may be enlarged with scalloped edges, may be a yellow coating or heat (red) in the middle jiao

6 heat in the stomach and retention of food in the stomach, stomach qi fails to descend due to perverse or rebellious stomach qi. This case illustrates two of the syndromes of qi — deficiency of qi and perverse or rebellious qi

7 invigorate the middle jiao to aid digestion and remove retention of food in stomach, subdue stomach heat, regulate the stomach qi and assist descent of the turbid qi

8 **Liangmen ST21** — treats epigastric distension and pain (due to stagnation of stomach qi), abdominal distension, vomiting, diarrhoea, poor appetite; used in preference to or combined with Zhongwan CV12; combine with Hegu LI4 for severe diarrhoea; combine with Neiting ST44 for burning sensation in the epigastrium and Liangqiu ST34 for acute apigastric pain

Tianshu ST25, front-mu point of large intestine — treats intestinal disorders, relieves food retention, clears heat and regulates qi; regulates the spleen and stomach; relieves mental irritation due to stomach disharmony (such as the heat of rebellious stomach qi)

Liangqiu ST34, xi-cleft point — harmonises the stomach, alleviates pain and treats acute conditions; combined with Liangmen ST21 also treats nausea, vomiting, belching and regurgitation

Zusanli ST36, he-sea point, earth point — harmonises the stomach, fortifies the spleen, resolves damp, clears fire, calms the shen and alleviates pain

Shangjuxu ST37, lower he-sea point, sea of blood point — regulates the function of stomach and intestines and transforms stagnation with direct action on large intestine; has the same function for the Large Intestine Channel as Zusanli ST36 has for the Stomach Channel

Fenglong ST40, luo-connecting point — allows connection with its biao li partner, spleen; resolves phlegm of any aetiology, clears phlegm from the heart and calms the spirit

Jiexi ST41, jing-river point, fire point — clears heat from the stomach, treats burning/stabbing epigastric pain, abdominal distension, belching and thirst

Chongyang ST42, yuan-source point — clears heat from the Stomach Channel, calms the shen

Neiting ST44, ying-spring point, water point — clears heat from the Stomach Channel, alleviates pain, resolves stagnant food, clears damp heat from the intestines and calms the shen

Lidui ST45, jing-well point, metal point — resolves stagnant food, clears heat, resolves fullness below the heart, calms the shen (insomnia); can prick the point to make it bleed

Hegu LI4, yuan-source point (LI) — powerful calming and antispasmodic action particularly for intestinal pain

Quchi LI11, he-sea point, earth point (LI) — relieves abdominal pain and distension; combine with Hegu LI4

Chapter 4 The Spleen Channel — Ms HT, 36 year old corporate consultant

1   internal, contributing lifestyle factors such as an irregular, poor diet, busy stressful job etc

2   –

3   a   deficiency; essentially a deficiency pattern (qi, blood, jin ye) even when poor transformation and transportation of jin ye lead to a local accumulation and excess of damp

    b   cold

    c   spleen, stomach

    d   Spleen, Stomach, Large Intestine and Lung Channels

4   normal rate, regular, empty, slippery spleen, deficient kidney

5   swollen body with teeth marks, pale or pink tongue proper, thin white coat over middle jiao and lower jiao

6   **ben** — spleen qi deficiency

    biao — damp accumulation (excess)

    wu xing — spleen failing to promote lung (qi and blood) in the generative cycle

7   strengthen and regulate spleen qi to transform and transport, disperse damp

8   **Taibai SP3**, yuan-source point — tonifies spleen, harmonises spleen and stomach, regulates qi and removes dampness; treats undigested food in the stool combined with Fuai SP16

    Gongsun SP4, luo-connecting point — strengthens spleen and middle jiao, resolves dampness, regulates qi, benefits the heart, calms the shen and regulates Chong Mai, stops diarrhoea and regulates the menstrual cycle

    Sanyinjiao SP6, meeting point of SP, LR & KI Channels — tonifies spleen qi, regulates spleen and stomach, resolves dampness, harmonises the liver, tonifies kidney, calms the shen and invigorates blood

    Daheng SP15 — strengthens spleen and large intestine and promotes their function; treats cold weak limbs, resolves dampness in the intestines particularly when there is mucus in the stool

    Tianshu ST25, front-mu point of large intestine — treats intestinal disorders, relieves food retention, clears heat and regulates qi; regulates the spleen and stomach; relieves mental irritation due to stomach disharmony (such as the heat of rebellious stomach qi)

    Zusanli ST36, he-sea point, earth point (ST) — harmonises the stomach, tonifies spleen qi, resolves damp, nourishes blood and yin, clears fire and calms the shen

    Shangjuxu ST37, lower he-sea point, sea of blood point (ST) — regulates the function of stomach and intestines and transforms stagnation with direct action on large intestine; has the same function for the Large Intestine Channel as Zusanli ST36 has for the Stomach Channel

    Fenglong ST40, luo-connecting point (ST) — allows connection with its biao li partner ,spleen; resolves phlegm of any aetiology, clears phlegm from the heart and calms the spirit

    Jiexi ST41, jing-river point, fire point (ST) — clears the heat from the stomach and channel, stimulates appetite, calms the shen

Neiting ST44, ying-spring point, water point (ST) — clears heat from the Stomach Channel, alleviates pain, resolves stagnant food, clears damp heat from the intestines and calms the shen

Hegu LI4, yuan-source point (LI) — powerful calming and antispasmodic action particularly for intestinal pain

Quchi LI11, he-sea point, earth point (LI) — relieves abdominal pain and distension; combine with Hegu LI4

Lieque LU7, luo-connecting point (LU) — regulates the water passages, opens and regulates Ren Mai

Taiyuan LU9, yuan-source point, shu-stream point (LU), influential point of vessels — strengthens lung qi and transforms phlegm, promotes the descending function of lung

Chapter 5 The Heart Channel — Miss DM, 17 year old schoolgirl preparing for scholarship exams

1   internal

2   –

3   a   deficiency — qi, xue, yin; may be accompanied by deficiency of kidney yin and hyperactive liver yang (excess)

    b   heat

    c   heart, spleen, lung

    d   Heart, Spleen, Stomach (knotted qi) and Lung Channels

4   rapid rate, regular, fine or thin, weak and thready

5   may be a midline crack reaching the tip, red tongue proper with red swollen tip, no coat

6   **ben** — [although the condition has arisen from Spleen and kidney qi xu, for the purpose of this exercise we are treating it as follows]

    biao — xin yin deficiency (deficiency fire)

    wu xing — hyperactive liver yang over-promoting heart in the shen cycle, failure of kidney water to warm and regulate heart on the Ko cycle

7   enrich heart yin, calm and pacify shen

8   **Lingdao HT4**, jing-river point, metal point — particularly good for controlling sweating in the upper body, especially the head; calms the spirit

    Tongli HT5, luo-connecting point — one of the main points to tonify heart, use in deficiency (xu) disorders; calms the spirit

    Yinxi HT6, xi-cleft point — regulates heart blood, moderates acute conditions, calms shen, disperses deficiency fire and alleviates night sweating

    Shenmen HT7, yuan-source point, earth point — tonifies heart and blood yin, pacifies the shen; useful to treat insomnia and agitation

    Shaofu HT8, ying-spring point, fire point — calms shen, regulates heart qi, calms heart fire

    Sanyinjiao SP6, meeting point of Spleen, Liver and Kidney Channels — tonifies yin, invigorates blood, calms the shen

    Zusanli ST36, he-sea point, earth point (ST) — harmonises the stomach, tonifies spleen qi, resolves damp, nourishes blood and yin, clears fire and calms the shen

    Neiting ST44, ying-spring point, water point (ST) — clears heat and fire from the Stomach Channel especially in the head and face, calms the spirit, treats nightmares

    Lieque LU7, luo-connecting point (LU), master point of Ren Mai — can be stimulated to release repressed emotions, treats emotional disorders, regulates the water passages, opens and regulates Ren Mai

    Taiyuan LU9, yuan-source point, shu-stream point (LU), influential point of vessels — strengthens lung qi and transforms phlegm, promotes the descending function of lung

Chapter 6 The Small Intestine Channel — Mr SB, 40 year old manager

1   external

2   a   cold

    b   wind

    c   acute — the condition may occur when degenerative changes are present in the neck, and if it is chronic it will be part of a Bi syndrome

3 –

4 initially 'normal' rate and rhythm, with time will become tense and superficial

5 may be 'normal' initially, a thin white coating may be present

6 acute invasion of wind cold

7 disperse the wind and the cold, restore the circulation of qi and blood in the affected channels

8 **Houxi SI3**, shu-stream point, wood point, master point of Du Mai — treats pain, stiffness and contracture, stiff neck, and muscles and tendons along the course of Du Mai. In clinic in Nanjing this was often the only point inserted (bilaterally) and the patient was told to move their neck while strong stimulation to the points was given

Yanglao SI6, xi-cleft point — moderates acute conditions, activates the channel and relieves pain, benefits the shoulder

Bingfeng SI 12 — expels wind and pain in the shoulder, scapula and neck

Ququan SI 13 — use for painful obstruction of the shoulder and scapula

Jianweishu SI 14 — important local point for painful neck and shoulder, expels wind and cold, activates the channel and relieves pain

Jianzhongshu SI 15 — activates the channel and relieves pain

Tianchuang SI16 — local point that activates the channel and relieves pain, regulates qi and calms shen

Lieque LU7, luo-connecting point (LU), master point of Ren Mai — benefits the head and nape of the head, use for stiff neck and shoulders and wind headaches, releases the exterior and expels wind, treats the initial stages of common cold

Hegu LI4, yuan-source point (LI) — powerful calming and antispasmodic action, treats pain along the channel, treats Bi syndrome

Shousanli LI10 — activates the channel and relieves pain, indicated for pain and immobility of the shoulder, alternate with Quchi LI11

Quchi LI11, he-sea point, earth point (LI) — activates the channel and relieves pain, treats Bi syndrome

[Luozhen, extra point — if using, use alone]

Moxa

Heat pack and massage

Chapter 7 The Bladder Channel — Miss SO, 22 year old office worker

1 external

2 **a** heat

  b dampness

  c acute

3 –

4 rapid, regular, slippery

5 tongue body red, yellow greasy moss over root of tongue

6 damp heat in the bladder

7 resolve dampness, clear heat, remove obstruction to the smooth flow of fluids in the lower jiao

8 **Pangguang BL28**, back-shu point of bladder — regulates the bladder and clears damp heat from the lower jiao

Weiyang BL39, lower he-sea point of San Jiao — regulates painful and difficult urination, relieves pain

Jinmen BL63, xi-cleft point — stops pain on urination, particularly in acute situations

Jinggu BL64, yuan-source point — clears heat (dysuria) from the bladder; calms the spirit

Zutonggu BL66, ying-spring and water point — clears heat from the bladder

Sanyinjiao SP6, meeting point of Spleen, Liver and Kidney Channels — resolves dampness in lower jiao, tonifies spleen, calms shen, activates the channel and relieves pain

Yinlingquan SP9, he-sea point, water point (SP) — regulates the spleen, resolves dampness, opens and regulates the water passages, and benefits the lower jiao

Quchi LI11, he-sea point, earth point (LI) — relieves abdominal pain and distension; combine with Hegu LI4

No moxa

Chapter 8 The Kidney Channel — Mr HB, 38 year old married computer consultant with two children

1   internal

2   –

3   **a**   deficiency, qi, yang, (xue xu)

   b   cold

   c   kidney, bladder, spleen, lung

   d   Kidney, Bladder, Spleen and Lung Channels

4   regular rate, tight, deep, weak; may be choppy if blood deficiency present

5   pale, scalloped, swollen, thin white coat

6   **ben** — injury and deficiency of jing and kidney qi with a decline in mingmen fire; over-thinking and fright cause injury to the heart and kidney

   biao — kidney yang deficiency

   wu xing — failure of spleen to promote lung (formation of blood and governing of qi) with failure of lung to promote kidney and spleen to control kidney

7   reinforce, restore and stabilise kidney yang, invigorate mingmen, nourish jing, promote blood, harmonise shen

8   **Taixi KI3**, shu-stream point, yuan-source point, earth point — tonifies kidney, harmonises the lower jiao, regulates urination, calms shen

   Dazhong KI4, luo-connecting point — reinforces kidney, anchors qi and benefits lung, strengthens will, dispels fear and stabilises emotions

   Shuiquan KI5, xi-cleft point — treats disorders of blood (all yin xi cleft points), moderates acute conditions and tonifies kidney

   Fuliu KI7, jing-river point, metal point — important tonification point of kidney, mother point of kidney water channel; strengthens the lumbar region

   Xinshu BL15, back-shu of heart — clears heart fire, calms shen, promotes sleep, tonifies and nourishes heart

   Pishu BL20, back-shu point of spleen — major point to tonify spleen and stomach function, nourishes blood, tonifies qi, resolves dampness; often combined with Shenshu BL23

   Shenshu BL23, back-shu point of kidney — tonifies kidney yang (moxa), regulates the water passages, reduces frequent urination and nocturia, strengthens lumbar area

   Zhishi BL52 — tonifies kidney, benefits jing, regulates urination, strengthens willpower, strengthens lumbar region

   Shenmen HT7, yuan-source, earth point (HT) — calms shen, promotes sleep, tonifies and nourishes heart

   Sanyinjiao SP6, meeting point of SP, LR & KI Channels — tonifies spleen qi, regulates spleen and stomach, resolves dampness, harmonises the liver, tonifies kidney, calms the shen and invigorates blood

   Yinlingquan SP9, he-sea point, water point (SP) — regulates the spleen, resolves dampness, opens and regulates the water passages, and benefits the lower jiao

   Zusanli ST36, he-sea point, earth point (ST) — harmonises the stomach, tonifies spleen qi, resolves damp, nourishes blood and Yin, clears fire and calms the shen

   Reinforcing technique

   Moxa is appropriate

Chapter 9 The Pericardium Channel — Mr CB, 46 year old warehouse manager

1   internal; the two main pericardium patterns are due to invasion by pathogenic heat and are relatively rare; consequently a heart syndrome has been chosen because it is more commonly seen in clinical practice

2   –

3   **a**   deficiency, excess — mixed syndrome, deficiency complicated by excess; qi, yang; stagnant blood, phlegm

   b   cold

   c   heart, pericardium

   d   Heart, Pericardium, Bladder, Spleen and Lung Channels

4   may be slowed, may be hesitant and intermittent, choppy or knotted, may be wiry — reflects stagnation of blood, pain associated with it, and aggravation by cold (tight)

5   purple tongue body, may have purple spots or purple tip, moist coating, distended sublingual veins

6   **ben** — heart yang deficiency

   biao — cardiac bi (xin xue yu shi, heart blood stagnation) complicated by phlegm

7   during attacks treat the biao, remove heart blood stasis and calm shen; between attacks treat the ben, invigorate heart yang to promote blood circulation and remove blood stasis, calm shen, warm spleen and kidney

8   **Quze PC3**, he-sea point, water point — treats pain along the channel, palpitations, cardiac pain, irritability and fear

   Ximen PC4, xi-cleft point — promotes circulation in the channels and collaterals of the chest to remove blood stagnation and pain, cools blood and stops bleeding; empirical point of arrhythmias, moderates acute heart disease and pain, specific for angina pectoris, pacifies shen

   Neiguan PC6, luo-connecting point, master point of Yin Wei Mai — regulates qi of Heart and Pericardium Channels, regulates heart blood and opens the chest, calms shen, clears heat, opens Yin Wei Mai

   Daling PC7, yuan-source point, xu-stream point, earth point — unbinds the chest, clears heat from the heart, cools the blood, calms the spirit

   Shuiquan KI5, xi-cleft point (KI) — treats disorders of blood (all yin xi-cleft points), moderates acute conditions and tonifies kidney

   Shencang KI25 — moves qi and blood in the chest, useful if heart yang deficiency is associated with kidney yang deficiency

   Dazhu BL11, influential point of bone, sea of blood point — use to nourish blood

   Jueyinshu BL14, back-shu point of pericardium — regulates heart blood, unbinds the chest, alleviates chest pain, palpitations and restlessness, reinforces yang

   Xinshu BL15, back-shu point of heart — calms the mind, tonifies and nourishes the heart, regulates heart qi and calms the spirit; use for chest pain such as angina where there is a sense of heaviness in the chest with restlessness

   Geshu BL17, influential point of blood — invigorates and moves blood, reduces phlegm, can moxa

   Shenshu BL23, back-shu point of kidney — tonifies kidney, regulates the water passages and benefits urination, fortifies yang, nourishes yin and jing; on the Ko cycle has a controlling action on the heart rate

   Shaohai HT3, he-sea point, water point (HT) — calms the shen, transforms phlegm and clears heat, moves stagnant blood

   Tongli HT5, luo-connecting point (HT) — one of the main points to tonify heart, use in deficiency (xu) disorders; calms the spirit

   Shenmen HT7, yuan-source point, shu-stream point (HT) — pacifies shen

   Xuehai SP10, — invigorates, regulates and moves stagnant blood, cools blood

   Taiyuan LU9, yuan-source point, shu-stream point (LU), influential point of vessels — strengthens lung qi and transforms phlegm, promotes the descending function of lung

   Disperse during an attack, even method between attacks

   Moxa is applicable if there is heart yang deficiency

Chapter 10 The San Jiao Channel — Mrs JC, 70 year old pensioner who lives alone

1   external

2   **a**   heat

   b   –

   c   acute — this is an acute injury with tissue damage and injury to muscles, tendons and ligaments of the wrist and forearm following trauma. Qi and blood stasis will occur in the local area and affected channels (LU, LI, HT, SI, PC, SJ). Recovery in an elderly person may be complicated by an underlying liver blood deficiency failing to nourish tendons and ligaments or external pathogen obstruction (painful Bi syndrome)

3   –

4   may be faster than normal, regular rhythm, the pulse shape will depend on any underlying deficiencies such as spleen and kidney qi deficiency of normal aging etc

5   initially normal for Mrs JC (take into account her age and health)

6   **ben** — injury to muscle, tendon and ligament following trauma, underlying blood deficiency (elderly)

   biao — qi stagnation and blood stasis in the affected channels (see above — 2c)

7   decrease pain by clearing qi stagnation and blood stasis and restoring normal flows of blood and qi in the affected channels, correct any underlying patterns of imbalance, calm shen

8   **Yangchi SJ4**, yuan-source point — relaxes tendons and ligaments, clears heat, alleviates pain, redness and swelling of the wrist

Waiguan SJ5, luo-connecting point, master point of Yang Wei Mai — clears heat, releases the exterior, activates the channel and alleviates pain, opens Yang Wei Mai

Zhigou SJ6, jing river and fire point — regulates qi and clears heat, activates the channel and relieves pain

Hegu LI4, yuan-source point (LI) — local point, activates the channel and relieves pain

Yangxi LI5, jing-river, fire point — clears heat, benefits the wrist joint, alleviates pain, calms shen

Houxi SI3, shu-stream, wood point (SI), master point of Du Mai — activates the channel and alleviates pain, clears heat, calms shen

Wangu SI4, yuan-source point (SI) — clears heat, reduces swelling, activates the channel and relieves pain

Yanggu SI5, jing-river, fire point (SI) — clears heat and reduces swelling, calms shen

Yanglao SI6, xi-cleft point (SI) — treats acute conditions, activates the channel, benefits the arm and relieves pain

Neiguan PC6, luo-connecting point (PC), master point of Yin Wei Mai — local point, clears heat

Daling PC7, shu-stream, yuan-source earth point (PC) — local point, clears heat, cools blood, calms shen

Tongli HT5, luo-connecting point (HT) — local point, activates the channel, relieves pain, calms shen

Shenmen HT7, shu-stream, yuan-source earth point (HT) — local point, relieves pain, calms shen

Shaofu HT8, ying-spring, fire point (HT) — activates the channel, clears heat, resolves pain, calms shen

Chize LU5, he-sea point, water point (LU) — makes lung qi descend, relaxes the tendons of the arm along the Lung Channel, local point for wrist pain and restricted movement

Taiyuan LU9, yuan-source point, shu-stream point (LU), influential point of vessels — strengthens lung qi and transforms phlegm, promotes the descending function of lung, local point

Yuji LU10, ying-spring point (LU), fire point — local point, clears heat along the Lung Channel

[Shangbaxie (extra) — for treatment of finger, hand and wrist injuries]

Chapter 11 The Gall Bladder Channel — Ms AB, 28 year old international flight attendant

1   internal

2   –

3   **a**   underlying deficiency leading to excess condition; qi; damp, phlegm, rebellious stomach qi

    b   heat

    c   spleen, gall bladder, middle jiao

    d   Spleen, Gall Bladder and San Jiao Channels

4   rapid rate, regular, slippery and wiry

5   swollen with teeth marks, red body, thick greasy yellow coating

6   **ben** — spleen qi deficiency

biao — damp heat in the gall bladder

wu xing — spleen qi deficiency resulting in accumulation of damp with inability to transform and transport nutrients, leading to dampness, spleen failing to promote lung (qi and blood), lung failing to control liver (Ko cycle)

7   disperse damp, clear heat in the gall bladder, stimulate smooth flow of liver qi and tonify spleen

8   **Riyue GB24**, front-mu point — benefits the gall bladder and spreads the liver qi, clears heat, harmonises the middle jiao, resolves damp heat

Dai mai GB26, master point of Dai Mai — drains dampness and treats pain in the lateral costal region

Yanglingquan GB34, he-sea and earth point — stimulates the liver qi and resolves dampness, activates the channel and relieves pain, clears gall bladder and liver damp heat; palpate Dannangxue, the extra point slightly below GB34, and needle if tender

Ganshu BL18, back-shu point of liver — spreads the liver qi, clears heat in the gall bladder, cools fire and clears damp heat

Danshu BL19, back-shu point of gall bladder — clears damp heat form the gall bladder and liver, clears pathogenic factors form Shaoyang, tonifies and regulates gall bladder qi

Pishu BL20, back-shu point of spleen — resolves dampness, tonifies spleen qi, regulates and harmonises the middle jiao

Zhigou SJ6, jing-river point, fire point (SJ) — clears heat in the three jiao and stimulates smooth flow of liver qi

Neiguan PC6, luo-connecting point (PC), master point of Yin Wei Mai — harmonises the stomach, alleviates nausea and vomiting, clears heat, opens Yin Wei Mai

Gongsun SP4, luo-connecting point (SP) — strengthens spleen and middle jiao, resolves dampness, regulates qi, benefits the heart, calms the shen and regulates Chong Mai, stops diarrhoea and regulates the menstrual cycle, pair as the master point of Chong Mai with Neiguan (master point of Yin Wei Mai)

Sanyinjiao SP6, meeting point of SP, LR & KI Channels — tonifies spleen qi, regulates spleen and stomach, resolves dampness, harmonises the liver, tonifies kidney, calms the shen and invigorates blood

Yinlingquan SP9, he-sea point, water point (SP) — regulates the spleen, resolves dampness, opens and regulates the water passages, and benefits the lower jiao

Quchi LI11, he-sea point, earth point (LI) — clears heat, cools the blood, drains damp and eliminates wind

Chapter 12 The Liver Channel — Ms VE, 25 year old planning a pregnancy

1   internal

2   –

3   **a**   excess, stagnant qi and blood, liver yang uprising

    b   heat

    c   liver, stomach, kidney, heart

    d   Liver, Pericardium, San Jiao and Gall Bladder Channels

4   normal rate, regular, wiry, may be choppy (if blood symptoms predominate)

5   normal tongue colour, may be petechiae along liver edges, thin yellow coating

6   **ben** — emotional imbalance or vexation

    biao — liver qi stagnation

7   regulate the menstrual cycle, nourish blood and qi, move stagnant liver qi, harmonise shen

8   **Taichong LR3**, yuan point, shu-stream point, earth point — invigorates liver, regulates liver and stops it invading spleen and stomach, spreads liver qi, subdues liver yang and extinguishes wind, nourishes liver blood and liver yin, regulates menstruation, disperses stagnant qi and blood and relieves pain, regulates the lower jiao, clears the head and eyes (menstrual migraine)

Zhangmen LR13, front-mu point of spleen, influential point of zang organs — regulates liver qi, harmonises liver and spleen, regulates middle and lower jiao, regulates circulation of qi and blood, strengthens the spleen, assists function of spleen to transform and transport nutrients

Qimen LR14, front-mu point of liver — treats pain in hypochondrium and breast region (in combination with Taichong LR3), invigorates blood, disperses masses, harmonises the liver and stomach

Yanglingquan GB34, he-sea point, earth point (GB) — activates the channel and relieves pain, spreads the liver qi, treats pain in the hypochondrium, clears liver and gall bladder damp heat

Zhigou SJ6, jing-river point, fire point (SJ) — regulates qi and clears heat in the three jiao, benefits the chest, used to treat pain in the chest and lateral costal regions, treats blockages of Ren Mai in women

Neiguan PC6, luo-connecting point (PC), master point of Yin Wei Mai — regulates the three jiao, regulates heart, calms shen, treats insomnia, unbinds the chest and regulates qi, harmonises stomach, alleviates nausea and vomiting, clears heat, opens Yin Wei Mai

Gongsun SP4, luo-connecting point (SP), master point of Chong Mai — tonifies spleen, harmonises middle jiao, regulates stomach and spleen and relieves pain, resolves dampness, calms shen, benefits heart and chest, regulates Chong Mai, treats gynaecological disorders

Gongsun SP4 + Neiguan PC6 — if female, needle Gongsun on the right foot and Neiguan on the left wrist (male left to right)

Diji SP8, xi-cleft point (SP) — regulates menstruation, invigorates blood, regulates the uterus, treats dysmenorrhoea (combine with Hegu LI4), harmonises the spleen and resolves dampness

Rugen ST18 — specific for breast pain and breast problems

Hegu LI4, yuan-source point (LI) — activates the channel and alleviates pain, combine with Diji SP8

Chapter 13 Ren mai — Ms LB, 28 year old business executive

1   internal

2   –

3   this is a mixed syndrome

    a   deficiency of qi and blood; stagnant blood, damp

    b   both cold and heat — qi deficiency leading to yang xu, however there are also features of blood heat (colour of menstrual flow)

    c   kidney, spleen, uterus, heart, liver

    d   Ren, Chong, Kidney, Spleen and Liver Channels

4   regular rhythm and rate; generally the pulse may be tight and thready, particularly in the kidney yin position

5   swollen and scalloped pink tongue body, white moss over middle and lower jiao, red tip, distended sub-lingual veins

6   **ben** — kidney and spleen deficiency

    biao — blood stasis

    wu xing — spleen failing to transform nutrients to make abundant qi and blood with lung failing to control liver on the Ko cycle

7   move qi and blood locally, dispel blood stasis and yet control heavy blood loss, nourish liver blood, protect and tonify spleen and kidney yang, harmonise shen

8   **Zhongji Ren3**, front-mu point of bladder — tonifies the bladder, connects with the uterus, and is one of the general tonification points for gynaecological diseases; combine with Guanyuan Ren4 to reinforce its action

    Guanyuan Ren4, front-mu point of small intestine — major tonification point, nourishes yang, reinforces qi and jing, regulates the uterus, nourishes blood, benefits yuan qi and tonifies kidney (receives a branch directly from kidney, and is connected to mingmen); powerful calming effect on the mind

    Qihai Ren6 — moves and supports qi, disperses stagnant qi (useful to treat abdominal pain due to stagnant qi, combine with Yanglingquan GB34), controls blood, tonifies spleen

    Zhongwan Ren12, front-mu point of stomach, influential point of fu — harmonises stomach and spleen, regulates stomach qi, tonifies the 'acquired qi', treats all spleen disorders of transformation and transportation; combine with Zusanli ST36 and Guanyuan Ren4

    Taichong LR3, yuan-source point, shu-stream point, earth point (LR) — invigorates liver, regulates liver and stops it invading spleen and stomach, spreads liver qi, subdues liver yang and extinguishes wind, nourishes liver blood and liver yin, regulates menstruation, disperses stagnant qi and blood and relieves pain, regulates the lower jiao, clears the head and eyes (menstrual migraine)

    Ligou LR5, luo-connecting point (LR) — spreads the liver qi, disperses stuck blood in the chest, treats disorders of genital and urinary areas, clears dampness and heat from the lower jiao, regulates menstruation, calms the spirit

    Daimai GB26, master point of Dai Mai — drains dampness and treats pain in the lateral costal region, regulates the uterus and menstruation, stops leucorrhoea and painful irregular periods

    Wushu GB27 — regulates Dai Mai, treats leucorrhoea and irregular menstruation, relieves lower abdominal pain, spreads the liver qi in the lower abdomen, regulates the lower jiao and transforms stagnation

    Weidao GB28 — similar indications and action as Wushu GB27

    Yanglingquan GB34, he-sea point, earth point (GB) — stimulates the liver qi and resolves dampness, activates the channel and relieves pain, clears gall bladder and liver damp heat; palpate Dannangxue, the extra point slightly below GB34, and needle if tender

    Jianshi PC5, jing-river point, metal point (PC) — regulates menstruation such as irregular, painful, clotted flow or leucorrhoea; moves liver qi and calms the mind

    Gongsun SP4, luo-connecting point (SP), master point of Chong Mai — tonifies spleen, harmonises middle jiao, regulates stomach and spleen and relieves pain, resolves dampness, calms shen, benefits heart and chest, regulates Chong Mai, treats gynaecological disorders

    Diji SP8, xi-cleft point (SP) — moderates acute conditions, regulates Qi and blood, regulates the uterus and menstruation, invigorates and removes blood stasis, stops pain during acute dysmenorrhoea and pre-menstrually in the treatment of chronic dysmenorrhoea (combine with Hegu LI4)

    Guilai ST29 — restores the uterus and genitals to normal, warms the uterus and lower jiao, treats vaginal discharge and menstrual problems related to blood stagnation

Qichong ST30, sea of water and grain point — precious relationship with Chong Mai and the uterus, regulates Qi and blood in the lower abdomen and genitals, use for leucorrhoea and painful menstruation

Reinforce the prescription with herbs that protect the kidney and spleen yang and break up blood stasis (be cautious and mindful of weak constitution when moving and breaking up blood stasis)

Chapter 14 Du Mai — Mr AF, 36 year old landscape gardener

1 internal

2 –

3 **a** deficiency of qi, blood, jing

   b cold

   c kidney, spleen

   d Du Mai, Kidney and Spleen Channels

4 the pulse will be deep, weak and slow, deficient kidney pulse (particularly kidney yang), slippery spleen pulse

5 pale tongue with scalloped edges, thin white coat (depending upon damp)

6 **ben** — kidney yang deficiency, spleen qi deficiency

   biao — qi and blood stasis in the affected back channels, with underlying blood deficiency

7 nourish kidney yang and strengthen the back, tonify jing, disperse cold, strengthen spleen function and harmonise shen

8 **Mingmen Du4** — treats stiffness of the spine, tonifies kidney yang (moxa), nourishes yuan qi and jing, strengthens the lower back and knees

   Dazhui Du14 — powerful meeting point of yang channels which transports the yang upward to the head and clears the mind, tonifies yang in deficiency conditions

   Baihui Du20, sea of marrow point — enlivens the mind, brightens the spirit, calms the shen, pacifies wind and subdues young, nourishes the sea of marrow, raises yang and treats prolapsed organs, particularly the rectum, uterus and vagina (moxa)

   Houxi SI3 and **Shenmai BL62**, master points that allow opening into Du Mai — tonify kidney, strengthen the back, boost willpower and lift depression. Needle Houxi on the left hand and Shenmai on the right foot (needle female right to left, male left to right)

   Guanyuan Ren4, front-mu point of small intestine — major tonification point, nourishes yang, reinforces qi and jing, regulates the uterus, nourishes blood, benefits yuan qi and tonifies kidney (receives a branch directly from kidney, and is connected to Mingmen); powerful calming effect on the mind

   Qihai Ren6 — moves and supports qi, disperses stagnant qi (useful to treat abdominal pain due to stagnant qi, combine with Yanglingquan GB34), controls blood, tonifies spleen

   Taixi KI3, shu-stream point, yuan-source point, earth point (KI) — tonifies kidney yang (moxa), harmonises the lower jiao, regulates urination, calms shen

   Zhaohai KI6, master point of Yin Qiao Mai — nourishes kidney yin and jing

   Pishu BL20, back-shu point of spleen — resolves dampness, tonifies spleen qi, regulates and harmonises the middle jiao

   Shenshu BL23, back-shu of kidney — strengthens the back, nourishes kidney jing, fortifies yang (moxa), nourishes yin, strengthens the lower back particularly in chronic back ache, resolves coldness and soreness in the lower back; combine with Zhishi BL52 to strengthen willpower, stimulate initiative and lift apathy; combine with Pishu BL20 to promote the formation of blood, benefits bones and marrow, regulates the water passages and benefits urination

   Guanyuanshu BL26 — local ah shi point for pain in region of the 5th lumbar vertebra, regulates the lower jiao

   Zhishi BL52 — tonifies kidney, benefits jing, regulates urination, strengthens the lumbar spine, strengthens sexual function and controls the discharge of semen, strengthens intention and willpower

   Shiqizhuixia, extra point — can be used as a local ah shi point for pain in the lumbar region

Chapter 15 The Other Six Extraordinary Vessels

Case	1st master point	2nd master point	Pair	Additional points
1	Gongsun SP4	Neiguan PC6	Chong Mai/Yin Wei Mai	Zhongwan Ren12 Tianshu ST25 Yinbai SP1 (moxa) Daheng SP15 Taixi KI3
2a*	Houxi SI3	Shenmai BL62	Du Mai/Yang Qiao Mai	Fengchi Du20 Sanyinjiao SP6 Fuliu KI7
2b	Zulingqi GB41	Waiguan SJ5	Dai Mai/Yang Wei Mai	Dazhui Du14 Fengchi GB20 Taixi KI3
3	Gongsun SP4	Neiguan PC6	Chong Mai/Yin Wei Mai	If deficient HT Yin, then Yinxi HT6 and Zhaohai KI6 (confluent)
4	Lieque LU7	Zhaohai KI6	Ren Mai/Yin Qiao Mai	Tiantu Ren22 Chize LU5
5	*Zulingqi GB41	Waiguan SJ5	Dai Mai/Yang Wei Mai	Fengchi GB20 Baihui Du20 Taichong LR3 Taixi KI3

*In clinical experience a superficial approach has proven more effective to relieve the headache. If the person with liver yang uprising is very kidney deficient, then working at a deeper level with Zulingqi/Waiguan sometimes appears to increase the headache because the liver yang is difficult to control.

Note: The extraordinary channels should be used with caution, especially in cases of qi and jing deficiency, and points to protect the kidney are advised in these situations.

Index